Spirit of Health

by
John Chamberlin

authorHOUSE™

1663 LIBERTY DRIVE, SUITE 200
BLOOMINGTON, INDIANA 47403
(800) 839-8640
WWW.AUTHORHOUSE.COM

First published by AuthorHouse 01/09/06

ISBN: 1-4259-1187-0 (e)
ISBN: 1-4208-7153-6 (sc)
ISBN: 1-4259-1186-2 (dj)

Printed in the United States of America
Bloomington, Indiana

This book is printed on acid-free paper.

Cover Kirlian Crystal Photo by Gene Falk

Disclaimer: This book is based on the opinions of John Douglas Chamberlin. They are not intended to replace a one on one relationship with a qualified health care professional and they are not intended as medical advice. They are intended as a sharing of knowledge and information from the research and experiences of John Chamberlin and his friends and fellow Alternate Healers. John Chamberlin encourages you to make your own health care decisions based upon your own research and with advice from a qualified health care professional.

Foreword

Rapid changes are occurring within our world today. We are experiencing extreme and devastating climatic events together with the appearance of diverse and strange diseases from varying and previously unknown origins. Most recently we have been exposed to terrorists who impose their will onto others, indiscriminately exploding devices as well as releasing chemicals to the wider population. We have no naturally established immune resistance to a resurgence of this cocktail of bacteria and viruses.

Whether we choose to acknowledge these threats to our health and well being or ignore them, the fact remains that we are all affected by them individually and globally. There is however good news, you can empower yourself and make a positive difference to you and your family now.

Spirit of Health is a book about the simple things that you can do when the medical system is paralysed and not able to offer you the best care and attention. The information I share with you in this book is a result of a lifetime journey of learning and experience in natural health at both a personal level and professionally through many years of private practice. This journey spans more than 20 years as a natural healer travelling and working in third world countries and participating in international healing expos; lecturing on health and healing; working with and guiding clients to find their own pathway back to well being on all levels by adopting a hands on and self help approach.

This self-help manuscript acts like a memory prodder for natural healing and triggers changes to all inner mind processes such as the negative disruptive conflicts of emotions, thoughts and words. The aim is to guide you to empower yourself and remove blocks and barriers causing disease that have been obstructing your inner health, peace, harmony and strength.

This book is written in layman terms but can also be used as a health therapist checklist for a professional health care giver to act upon. Included in the text is information on low cost natural pain relieving therapies, aromatherapy oils, herbs, gem stones, color and its effects. Information is given on environmental checks and explanations that are easily assimilated so that a stressed person can make informed decisions and choices about their own actions and environments or find the right professional who can help.

Informed readers can choose to take their personal power back and be responsible for their own health and emotional security to enjoy renewed energy and joy. Instead of accepting the shame blame or DNA patterns from family inheritance, condemning the boss, government, God, Universal Intelligence, etc. they can now gain understanding and insight into their role of accepting disease in their lives and consequently commence the healing process. Readers can now choose to acquire and embrace health with passion!

My wish is that you find answers to most of your questions and find peace within. I thank and embrace all of my teachers, loved ones, family and friends who encouraged me along this journey "to be of service".

In Light, Love and Joy.   John

The author acknowledges that he has an eclectic mind and picks up information at times when directed, assimilates the information and does not recall at times where this information was from as most have been obtained when travelling the world. In his own quest for health and healing for a pain free joy filled life he has gained information from many different seminars and from many different teachers, from children, newspapers, seminar leaders and the Internet but has proven them all to his satisfaction in private practice.

To his teachers and mentors either living or in spirit he is eternally grateful and gives thanks.

If there is any information printed following that may be from original material, that may have been copyrighted before or after he received the information and your name is not attached with the appropriate creditation please accept his apology. Should you contact the author or the publishers the appropriate notation will be made on acceptance of this proven advice as we have tried to give credit where credit is due. In his opinion this book is a collection of some of the most simple mind joggers but can be profound dynamic life changing procedures. If you contributed in any way there are hundreds of people who have had life changes for the positive and will be today be sending you blessings for your contribution. Thank you for using your energy to purchase this book as a percentage of the proceeds will go to helping people who are less fortunate than us to have operations and healings. Readers please understand that for practical purposes both sexes are referred to when "he" is used in the text, and no discrimination or disparity is intended.

Table of Contents

Introduction

Sound, pristine health is a blessing that money cannot buy!
Restore, reconcile, and value your health today.
This is a book about taking charge of your own LIFE and cure DIS-EASE. This does not necessarily mean life threatening, however if you are sick or not well in any shape or form then it is time to take charge of your own emotions, mind and body and do something about it.

Many people say they are dying with cancer or with AIDS, etc. They are not! They are living with a dis-ease, that right up to the last minute of death can have a reprieve. Miracles do happen and it is not our right to give someone a death sentence by saying they are dying with this or that.

Don't buy this book unless you are prepared to make the commitment and dedication to at least finish reading this book, follow the simple non-costly directions and take the road back to strength and vigour. It is your God given right to have health, or at least feel better about yourself within a short time.

The responsibility starts and ends with you! No one else is responsible for you, not your mother, father, family, doctor, health practitioner, government or situations you have been in. **No one but you! And the sooner you accept this as a fact of life, the quicker the change towards better health in your life will be. Choose to take your health power back for quality of life.**

It is absolutely irresponsible to expect the government or some such body to be in a caretaking position, to be there for you and make all your decisions regarding your health. Most therapists know and firmly believe that if more people took responsibility for their own lives there would be a lot less friction going on in the world, and this planet would be a better place to live on.

If you are in the business of trumping up charges just to make your life easier, cheating on anyone, suing people, taking money

1

surreptitiously from a government or employer however justified in your conscious mind, then you have no right to expect a quality of life as your own subconscious mind will not allow it. Make the changes to truth now! It is never impossible, nor are you too old to change!

Life is a school, and is not meant to be perfect all the time for this is a beautiful but imperfect planet. When life becomes perfect, it is time for us to leave planet Earth. So why do you want to leave this planet in so much of a hurry? To see how we are able to handle living on this planet here, there are tests, a word I dislike, to see how we handle life, and if we have to learn a lesson again, we will. Maybe we didn't learn it the first time through. Circles are really more easily seen and prevalent in and around a practicing relationship.

Pain is a teacher, a warning, and a choice to go ahead or stop, whether emotional, mental, physical or spiritual. Emotion is energy in motion and is used for us to feel and digest what is happening. When we are too stressed or occupied in doing things and not listening to the warning signs, we will miss the body and emotions' greatest warning signals.

When creating our human body God gave us two ears and one mouth. It is a shame that most people don't take the inference and listen twice as much as they speak.

If we spent our lives listening twice as much as speaking superfluous gossiping words and criticism and conserved and directed that wasted energy into helping others, this world would be a better place. To gossip and put someone else down has a negative on ourselves and have been proven using kinesiology, body electrics and body harmony. Speaking negatively or having negative thoughts weakens **the gossip's** body and emotions. When we feel the need to gossip in an attempt to feel better about ourselves we have really poor self-images and put others down to make us feel better when they squirm. Who do you know who is like this? Avoid them!

This book may challenge your beliefs, help you to think about things you may not want to remember, get you to experience healing modes that may put you on the edge of your seat of uncomfortability, test your courage and help you to re-experience parts of your lifetime you may not want to remember.

It's a proven fact! Should you not want or wish to remember parts of your life, or areas of your life are blank and there is no memory, the subconscious mind must be protecting you from these memories. This will be affecting your health, holding you back from a healthy and happy life mistakenly thinking it is helping you.

This does not in any way suggest that it may be something bad or horrible but more likely there is a lack of understanding by the subconscious mind. This in turn may be stopping us from having all the good things in life, as the subconscious views of perception have been drawn from a distorted child's point of view without an adult perception or overall view.

If you are looking for an intellectual answer to all your problems, you will be lucky to find it in this book as I and many others in the healing professions know that in order to be well, happy and healthy **You have to feel it to heal it!**

COMMUNICATION AND MIRRORS

Know that if you are not comfortable to talk openly about yourself in all situations, your problem has a hold on you. When life has a hold of your heart and emotions, its pathway is effecting your energies in a negative way.

Take responsibility for your part in the so-called bad/traumatic areas of your life now, forgive yourself for your part in it, forgive others for not being there for you in your hour of need and ease the burden. Know that the mere fact you are alive today means you obviously have had a lot of strength to still be here, as a lot have not had that strength, gave up and didn't make it.
Acknowledge yourself now for having the strength to carry on!

John Chamberlin

NEVER REGRET GROWING OLDER. IT'S A PRIVILEGE DENIED TO MANY!
(Old Indian Proverb)

There is no bad or good in the subconscious mind, there is just what is, what we have come to learn in the school of life and what one learns from the pathway's situation.

Emotions are something else as our control issues and egos come into it.

RELATIONSHIPS Every person is a Mirror.

Our original state of life is one of wholeness, joy, spontaneity, love, peace, and harmony, connecting with one another and welcoming life as core energy. Being vulnerable without losing anything of ourselves but rather empowering ourselves by the union with another.

Our deep-seated biological roots for survival is a search for contact and relationship with others.

Though we think we choose a partner consciously, the primary choice is and lays with the subconscious mind's desire to complete or correct what was not completed from childhood. We normally select a partner who was wounded in the same adapted areas and carries both negative and positive characteristics.

Know that relationship is for healing each other and nothing ever gets hurt except our ego. Through our emotions/private space thought we have been invaded by conditioning from others that we have adapted as our own. As well we have been subconsciously programmed from the womb and have been wounded at various stages of development in childhood through over/under parenting skills that are the result of our parents' and society's wounds and/or external situational stresses and predators.

These patterns normally kick in when our conditional love is being threatened and the other person is breaking the control of our expectations of what we believe to be the right way. We believe that person under our acquired rules for living is not free to experience

4

life as they wish. There is a universal law however, that the more a person holds on and pulls to control another, universal power will push the person away with greater force. It is easier to just let go, be in the moment, experience your partner's uniqueness and prepare ourselves to be vulnerable and **Intimate**. Intimate really means, **into me I see.**

A key to relationships is to always speak our truth as this allows each party to know what is going on and so feel a measure of safety in this fact. Remember lying by omission is still lying.

The inner child of us needs to be nurtured by the so called big person within us so we are dealing with safety and unsafety and often see or get the urge to run away to the greener grass on the other hill. Someone else will always understand, without having the old conditioning of living with you it is fresh knowledge, new and challenging. The other avoidance is to emotionally withdraw which often means not being there for the respective partner or going to our castles and caves, and being really mystical and magical but not in reality, leaving emotionally while our bodies are still there.

In doing couple therapy after each partner has had prior sessions with me we hear some surprises. Time and again we get from one partner or the other, You never told me that and I had no idea that you felt that way about that. Why didn't you tell me? Communication development is so very important and the truth sometimes hurts, but to stay in denial is fooling yourself that everything is OK when it isn't.

A really good way to face certain situations that happened in my life was to ask the question of why?

1. Why did I draw this situation into my life?
2. What am I learning from this?
3. Do I chose to stay in this situation? If I do will I benefit from the experience?

4. Is there anything that I need to choose to do to change this situation? Positively!
5. Is it best for all concerned for me to just walk away from it, or will only make things worse? It takes more courage to walk away from a fight and stay peaceful than go through it.

If you are upset ask;

1. Why did I draw this person into my path?
2. What am I to learn from this?
3. What is this person mirroring to me?
4. Does this person remind me of someone else who I have not forgiven?
5. Is this person doing something that in my perception of life is not in my moral code or upbringing?
6. Is my reaction a form of anger that I never got away with so why should they? (Judgment)
7. Does this person reflect to me how I would really like to be and I am jealous?
8. Is it important enough in the reality of my life for me to stay in this situation, or them to stay in my presence?
9. If my life ended tomorrow, would this really matter enough for me to get upset about?

If I am upset **it is my problem** and I can get over it or leave or change the situation. No one is responsible for my feelings, thoughts, or emotions.
I AM IN CHARGE OF ME. PERIOD!

It is so important to state your true feelings and emotions and yet not be physically violent.
To never feel anger means that you will never feel love or passion for life.

Anger is an emotion too and can cause horrendous dis-ease in our systems. Passion can be misconstrued as anger. If we had an incredible amount of anger in our childhood we may also negatively react towards someone who is passionate about the truth and misconstrue it as anger or control from the person, especially if as growing up we were subjected to anger as manipulation.

Let me share one of the greatest truths given to me on holding/squashing down anger.

In my mind, it was not appropriate to speak to the person concerned, in case it may hurt her feelings. I was feeling really hurt and like Jesus, felt that I was carrying the cross and could not handle the stress and strain. At the same time I was not aware of the building up of stress in my body. Feeling hurt, pain racking through my body, knowing my partner was sick and had enough of her own problems to deal with, I should be strong enough and man enough to deal with this. I was unknowingly stuffing down all my feelings and emotions, so as well as the emotional pain, the communication and intimacy in our relationship really sucked.

In the midst of a meditation a voice said to me, What makes you think you're better than God?

I replied that I was not but I was working on trying to be a good person and by stating what I really felt, would only make matters worse. The voice said, Could it be much worse? I stated Not much so the reply was So you think you are better than God then.

At this I was starting to get angry at the voice. I believed that statement was foreign to me and totally unacceptable, as I would never compare myself to God.

The voice said again, Well didn't God get angry and flood the world once?

And did not Jesus get angry and throw the money lenders out of the temple?

What makes you better than God by stating it's not OK to get angry.

If God and Jesus, with all the wisdom and knowledge that they have felt it necessary to be angry, to let out the negative feelings and injustices, then you have that right also!

I was really humbled and have to this day expressed when I was not happy with a situation and my health improved immediately. You have the right to feel your own anger, feelings, emotions but do not have the right to control, manipulate or hurt anyone else by you expressing that anger.

Dr Barbara DeAngelis in her relationship seminars **Secrets For Making Love Work** (highly recommended) talks of people emotionally taking energy from their partner. Emotionally and energetically we are like two tanks with water in them, connected to each other at the bottom. When one partner gets emotionally down then the other partner or family member helps fill them up with caring and love. Your family is linked by your love, or by your loving the person intimately usually at the heart and base energy centers. This also means that when a partner stuffs their feelings it forces the other partner or a member of the family to express it for them, through the energetic connections. In my experience when a partner is angry and upset it is time for me to ask myself what part of my feelings of hurt, frustration and anger am I not expressing.

Barbara's book on **How To Make Love All The Time** is a must for relationships and can be read together for the Ah Ha syndrome. The write yourself a love letter on page 124 in her book is a wonderful way to find out where you are in life and why you are angry with family.

NOTE WELL! What anger or negative emotions you repress, your partner, children, or loved one will express for you.

Either your partner or other members of the family will express what you repress. If it is not, then your own body mind and emotions will be like an angry boil waiting to erupt in festering anger or dis-ease.

A good way to get to the bottom of a problem within yourself if you are not sure of where your stress is coming from, is to imagine in your mind's eye a gauge similar to a car petrol/gas gauge. See numbers 1-2-3-4-5-6-7-8-9-10 running left to right, with 10 indicating the highest stress level. An arrow underneath this points to the numbers just like a fuel gauge. Bring up behind the gauge each person in your family one by one and all the things that are annoying you about that person and then let your mind give you a stress number.

Sometimes I am really surprised at the stress level of an issue that I am in denial over. This gauge can be used at work and for a lot of different things. It also gives a person a place to work from to release relationship stress.

Do you know that a **ninety-five per cent of what we fear never happens?** What a waste of energy it is to worry!

FEAR equals FALSE EVIDENCE APPEARING REAL equals FORGET EVERYTHING AND RUN
FEARS opposite word equals REJOICE. Look for a door to FREEDOM AND JOY in Health.

> **One needs to risk everything to be fully alive, a total commitment to moment of now, to have FREEDOM.**

In most of the counseling situations we find where a partner is seemingly happy at work, and on getting home finds themselves unhappy and irritable, then someone in the family unit is suppressing. It is a known fact now that when children's food intake is being watched they still become extremely hyperactive and angry for no seemingly good reason. The counselor's need to talk to the parents of the child to find out who is suppressing feelings and emotions that are being expressed by the child.

If you are not happy, feeling anger about a situation, you have the right to state that you are not happy with ___THE PROBLEM__ _and that you wish to talk about it. You wish to communicate, be heard and not be shut down. If any violence is threatened or used then the plot is lost, and professional help will be needed and a place of safety chosen to communicate.

Most times it is enough to state, I am really angry about this situation, and while I am not going to do anything about it as I do care for you and for our relationship, I need to go for a walk, cool down and think about this. I will be back at approximately _____ am/pm. This gives time to cool off and not say or do things that may hurt each other.

9

If the hurts have cooled by the time you get back, fine, but if not you then need to choose whether or not you need more time to think it through, so the following suggestions may help.

1. I choose not to talk about this _____(subject) until _____ (whenever.) or
2. When can we talk this problem through to find a solution, as I am still not happy as this problem is still intolerable for me, or I do not blame you and am looking for resolution.
3. I do not want to or wish to discuss anything now as I am still too upset and I treasure our relationship and you or I do not wish my thinking to be clouded by saying something that is too emotional right now.
4. When can we do this? How about 3 o clock tomorrow, does that suit? Get a time and keep it, and if you think the meeting could be a really explosive situation meet in a public place or in a therapist's office to keep the situation calm.

Most times silly little arguments are used just to get the attention of the other partner so if this is happening maybe it is time to look at holding the person nitpicking at you.

The words "I agree to disagree" will most times shut down a conversation going nowhere.
When asked what do you mean then say, I agree that you are right in what you are thinking but no amount of convincing or talking will get me to agree with what you believe, so let's forget this conversation and get back to loving each other now. I respect you and love you for your uniqueness. Want a cup of tea or coffee? Change the conversation now!

Assure and get a nurturing hug from the person before retiring or leaving if possible, so they know that you care. Except in violent situations.

Ever wondered why contact sports and lifting weights are so popular? Sports like wrestling, football, etc. where people get so involved and literally spew angry words at the players as though their life depended on it. The relief afterwards comes from shouting out the tension inside created from the frustration's about their life.

With the financial and emotional pressures that are put on the modern couple, and for all the violence, emotional blackmail and immoral conditioning on our TVs it is a wonder any people are together at all because it takes much courage and patience. The rewards however are great and I believe the road to accelerated personal growth/ awareness is in relationships! It's too easy to hide.

A good exercise to find out what conditioning we may be carrying in our bodies in the cellular DNA/RNA from our relatives and giving to our children, is to take a large sheet of paper, write your name in the middle and under this write all your positive and negative traits and illnesses and pains.

If you are not sure of your own personality positives and negatives, write down on a separate piece of paper the names of five of your friends and all their positives and negatives. Circle all the same traits in your friends and these will be yours also, if you are really honest.
Birds of a feather gather together?

Then above your name write out all your family tree with the names of your mother, father, uncles and aunts with brothers and sisters on the same line as yourself if applicable. Above your parents write out grandparents, their brothers and sisters and then dig in to find out all about them. Successful, poor, angry, happy sick, well, comic, good relationship, bad relationship, diseases, died of, etc. Gather any little bit of information you can get no matter how small and insignificant it may seem. Take your time and at the end of this a pattern will emerge of the issues that are passed down from generation to generation. If you have had children add their names under yours and add all their personality traits and aches and pains.

John Chamberlin

When this is all completed, circle all the words that keep repeating. It's also scary to see what patterns reappear in your children. Your paper should end up similar to looking like this.

Great Grandpa (Paternal)
Positives Negatives Illnesses Died Of?

Great Grandma (Maternal)
Positives Negatives Illnesses Died Of?

Grandfather
Positives Negatives Illnesses Died Of?

Grandmother
Positives Negatives Illnesses Died Of?

Great Uncles
Positives Negatives Illnesses Died Of?

Great Aunts
Positives Negatives Illnesses Died Of?

Father
Positives Negatives Illnesses

Mother
Positives Negatives Illnesses Died Of?

Uncles
Positives Negatives Illnesses

Aunts
Positives Negatives Illnesses Died Of?

You
Positives Negatives Aches Pains

Brothers
Positives Negatives Illnesses

Sisters
Positives Negatives Illnesses

Children
Positives Negatives Illnesses   Positives Negatives Illnesses

Look for the recurring patterns and concentrate on making changes in these directions in both you and your children.

The Behavioural Barometer

When we are challenged by verbal abuse / anger in our younger years, when feeling we have no protector/s, sometimes we will blank out and look away from the perpetrators. We lock certain negative words in our subconscious with our eyes and remove a part of our spirit to somewhere else in the universe as we feel deserted and sometimes self punish ourselves every time certain words are said.

What these words really mean by Gordon Stokes /Daniel Whiteside in their book called The Behavioural Barometer gives really deep insight into some of the word blocks that are emotionally charged within the different levels of the mind depending on our individual experience of life. You need to be trained in this, but it does not take long. It really is amazing what words get stuck in our head so to speak with emotion behind this. Well worth a session or two as I have seen grown men brought to their knees as they access their subconscious mind for release.

Soul retrieval, soul fragmentation, the emotional barometer and regressional therapies combine excellently to allow our spirit to come back to the one power charged oneness we once were

SEX. Dare I mention this?

Now that I have your attention, as a guy I have a message for all of you. In all the therapies that deal in the subconscious mind with people who have sexual problems it has been proven to me beyond doubt that the female of the human species controls sexuality. If we look at the number of floors of women's clothing/accessories/appliances in retail stores compared to the small spaces that men have to purchase clothes it is obvious to me also that woman holds all the power too.

We fellas obviously thought we were in charge by being the stronger species, the protectors, and most women allowed this for them to feel safe and to have someone around to do all the heavy work. Similar to slave labor.

Not being happy with that, the female of the species has now entered the work force and is trying to emulate the male species which is totally against her femininity and so usually to cope, she becomes more ruthless than the men who previously screwed up.

Don't copy the males who were our predecessors girls as they were not sensitive enough to do it right. Be aware of the new order of male who can accept you for who you are, be loving and nurturing and does not nor will accept to be put down. Both human male and female have made horrendous mistakes but know women hold the power of sexuality and we guys trail along like little puppets most of the time. Your sisters need a little more integrity also to help with the peace in the world. Although DNA testing will start to keep them honest.

What I am getting at is this. We guys do not choose a woman as they choose us. I have yet to see a guy resist a woman who is really in love with him and has chosen him as her own, as his whole mind becomes like mush and his head will not think about anything else until he calls and does something about it. We males just think we did the choosing.

Energetically speaking, when a couple make love, when the penis is inserted, the energies of the auras are joined and become one. When ejaculation takes place, ignition takes place through all the energy centers starting at the base center and continues all the way up the bodies that are lying together face to face. This is why a single masturbation is very unfulfilling for most as there is no blending of male and female energies and usually a void.

With each center igniting the energy is shot upwards to the next center until the crown center ignites. At this point a clairvoyant can see the two souls come out of the bodies and entangle and enmesh with the female taking and balancing the male energies she is needing to balance within her. The male takes and balances the female energies he needs to balance within him. At this time of total balance of both the male and female energies we can connect to our source really easily. After the tide of passion is over the male is normally quiet and usually wants to take a small cat nap and usually loses his erection for a short time until he comes back into his male energy again and finds his erection again. Having acquired a male energy, the girls will normally be full of the more aggressive energy and will want to talk and not want the male to sleep.

Anyone who studies **Tantric Sex** will find these problems alleviated with practice, as it is a fallacy that a guy will lose his erection after ejaculation. He can if he chooses to go on making love for hours as long as the desire is there with the woman of his choice still wanting that stimulation. However if the woman believes a guy after ejaculation will go soft, the male will loose all stiffness even though he may want to have more fun. The male is conditioned not to hurt his lady sexually as this obviously would cut off the supply of intimacy and sex. Woman hurt, no loving.

If a woman has an infection in the vaginal area or is sore or uncomfortable for any reason, any sensitive guy loses his erection in a matter of seconds after sensing the hurt, even though he may be frustrated.

There are guys who are rough and like getting back through their partner at some woman who has hurt them before, and even girls who like to play rough with their man to get back at their prior predator. Not all of these power plays are conscious decisions.

When a woman has a baby, there is a lot of fear before and afterwards if they will be OK sexually and if they will be tight enough in the virginal area for their man. She makes the mistake of pushing out her sensual energies or bearing down to try and be tighter for the experience. After a baby or a thrush/candida experience when the private parts have been hurt very badly a lot of women develop muscles so tight they can become almost inpenetratable. Especially with the subconscious mind recognizing the hurt and mistakenly saying to have sex means to be hurt so we will stop that energy now.

Fear of being hurt is natural and to be hurt a lot in the reproductory areas usually ends up with the woman energetically pushing away the sexual energy so her partner has week erections or can be really strong and will go weak just before penetration. This partner will normally find no trouble however with another partner who is keen to make love and finds him desirable. It is usually undesirable for the male to even try this in case the humiliation returns and he can't do it as his ego has been hurt.

Many times when this happens it can be alleviated if the lady is deprogrammed of all her bad experiences in hypnosis and given a self hypnosis exercise to do of sensing/seeing herself experiencing the intimate sexual act with her partner, how she would like her climax to go and how she would like her body to react during the experience. The next time the urge comes she needs to concentrate on bringing her partner's wand of light into her sacred space. By her concentration and picturing /sensing all of her muscles pulling in, this will activate a wave like action in the womb and vaginal area and will pull the walls in much tighter than before extending the erectional staying power of the male to the delight of both. Experiencing the light energy inside her without movement and without pain at times also will do wonders for both of the partners for a change and will enhance sensitivity.

Then we sometimes get a partner who is complaining of his or her partner not wanting to have sex with them. It is amazing how many times after being asked by the therapist, "when did you cheat on your partner then?" The embarrassed reply is usually the time his/her partner closed down sexually.

So many people today are having extra marital lovemaking and think they are getting away with it. Let me tell you that **everything is known to the subconscious mind and so if you do cheat, expect your own subconscious mind to tell your partner the whole truth in MIRROR TALK.**

Consciously the partner may not know about your affairs or may be in denial for security sake. The partner may also be confused, not know why he or she have become cold with shut down sexual feelings and don't have that trust towards you any more.

A classic example was using a Mirror Talk machine that plays a voice recording backwards at different speeds. This machine has proven that when we consciously talk to someone our subconscious talks backwards to the same person telling them the whole truth and nothing but the truth. Scary for cheating lying people huh!

In a recording I have heard the voices of four friends who decided to play their voices backwards to see what their subconscious minds were saying to each other. When the husband and wife of the friends spoke together his subconscious mind said he had been unfaithful on his latest business trip and when asked by his wife if this was true he denied it. Two days later the whole truth came out and the marriage was saved but the husband recognized the need for the total truth especially now as his wife bought a new Mirror Talk machine.

Another big NO in relationships is to use sexuality for gain. Time and again I have heard a woman say she was not going to have sex with her husband because he would not agree or wouldn't buy such and such for her or her family. Take it from me, this is absolutely stupid on the part of anyone who uses this practice. Firstly, why would you deny your own body pleasure and secondly, to make love for gain on any level puts you in the same category of a prostitute or a pimp as you are selling your body. Thirdly, it is a well-known conditioning fact that if men do not have sex for a long time they will get aggressive and angry or leave you for another so to withhold will only make this situation worse. Keep your disagreements out of the bedroom!

Masturbation is another gray area for the subconscious mind as it is not the real thing and quite often I hear complaints of no one is ever able to satisfy me as I can myself, and so I masturbate. If your choice is to masturbate then that is your choice to avoid intimacy, but know that no one will know all your choice spots/erogenous zones as much as you do, unless you are willing to share these with the person you are with.

Don't expect everyone to be a mind reader either. He or she may be just like you at this moment and feeling very vulnerable. To use a vibrator without asking your partner beforehand is also considered very bad manners and a put down to most males who do not compare themselves to a machine even when they tell you otherwise.

How would you like it if he brought in his blow up dolly to help out after you have had enough? Not good practice for loving relationships. To masturbate a lot also dissipates the attracting energies of attracting a mate to you, so get ready for a lonely life.

When we get horny we send an energy out to the world that I am ready to meet and mate so sometimes it is better to go with a frustrating flow for a while and let the attracting energies go to work.

If you have in your mind no choice but to masturbate, then I suggest you put on several candles and create a sacred space around you. In your mind create and surround yourself with a pink bubble from the universe before commencing and this will stop any earthbound spirits attaching to you on astral body. Pink is universal love.

SACRED SEX II the video is highly recommended for sexual therapy where the film shows a beautiful way of setting up a sacred space for love making and gives practical explanations of love making and is very tastefully done.
It can be hired at most video stores.

Here is something to remember if you always work/play to please your partner when making love. Allow yourself to be intimate and risk being vulnerable, find out what he or she likes and give without thought of pleasing yourself. You will always be satisfied and happy sharing sexual experiences with a caring partner.

If you don't ask, it's always a NO! What can you lose? You may be pleasantly surprised.

Most people know what they don't want, but haven't expressed what they do want to the world and universe.

What do you want in your life for **you**? Not what your children, mother, father, loved one, etc., wants.

WHAT DO YOU WANT? Remember free choice! By writing out what you do want out of life will focus your sixty billion brain cells into action!

Maybe I want to be successful.
I want to be loved.
I want and wish to be well paid, rewarded and recognized.
I want perfect health.
I want a beautiful spiritual person to share my life with.
I want to be one with my source.
I want zero pain in my body, mind and emotions.
I want there to be no pain, starvation or suffering in the world.

Life is a puzzle. A puzzle is a challenge and we love a challenge. The pieces will fit and the pieces are all here. We just have to have the will to challenge life back to dare your life and health to get out of line!

Risk!

To laugh is to risk appearing the fool.
To weep is to risk being called sentimental.
To reach out to another is to risk showing your true self.
To place your ideas and dreams before the crowd is to risk being called naive.
To love is to risk not being loved in return.
To live is to risk dying.
To hope is to risk despair.
To try is to risk failure.

But risks must be taken, because the greatest risk in life is to risk nothing.

The people who risk nothing do nothing and become nothing.

They may avoid suffering and sorrow but they simply cannot learn to feel, and change, and grow, and love, and live...

Chained by their servitude, they are slaves, they have forfeited their freedom.

Only people who risk are truly free.

Author Unknown

HUGS are so important to good health and according to all the experts we need about 20 hugs a day. I am talking about non-sexual, non-confrontational hugs and think the following sums it up beautifully:

Have a hug because hugs are not only nice they are needed. Hugs can help relieve pain and depression, make the healthy healthier and the most secure among us even more so. Hugging feels good, overcomes fears, eases tension, provides stretching exercises if you are short, provides bending and stooping exercise if you are tall. Hugging does not upset the environment, saves heat, is portable, requires no special equipment, makes happy days happier, makes impossible days possible. (Author Unknown)

I can already hear some of you saying "but I can't do that as it is not safe," and in some really rare situations that is true. When I was teaching self healing training with some girls in Australia on how to be open and vulnerable, still remain in their femininity and not give their power away, this question came up.

One girl said to give hugs was really impossible as whenever she hugged someone she usually ended up in bed making love whether she really wanted to or not. She felt responsible for past boyfriend's reactions. This is what she was taught by her mother who felt a woman should be responsible for a guy's feelings, so this question fell into a lively discussion, with me thinking why wasn't she around me when I was younger?

It was suggested to her that the next time she went out she hugged the person if she felt safe. If the person started to move or gyrate against her she could break the hold by slapping him on the back fairly hard with one hand and then using her other hand place against the man's chest just under his neck and push firmly away. Look directly into his eyes and say gently and quietly so no one could overhear but with power and conviction. This was not what she wanted from him and this relationship at this point of time. She liked to hug people, and if he ever gyrated or tried sexual moves again she would never hug him again. She would still be continuing to hug her other friends. If she wanted to change the situation she would discuss this with him. "So what is it to be?" She had to be firmly resolved in her mind about this and not change her mind even a little bit.

When she did this the guy smiled a little sheepishly and said that she didn't mean it, he hoped, and he couldn't be blamed for trying. On her reaffirming she did mean it, she had no trouble with this unacceptable behavior again as she had formed in her aura that she liked to hug, and no one was going to spoil it for her even though he was cute and good looking. She also had another guy who tried to do this to her again after she asked him not too. She refused to hug him again and regained her power and self respect back and called me at three o clock in the morning to say that it worked.

If someone else cannot handle you being open and friendly without sexual connotations, then it is their problem, as long as you have not been teasing and leading them on.

When hugging a person who pats you on the back, do you know what the body language for that means? They are trying to shut down your, sexual feelings towards them, or are afraid of their own feelings. Interesting huh?

HUGS are fun. Do it, take the risk of hugging at least among your friends.

There is no such thing as a bad hug, only good ones and great ones. They are not fattening and they don't cause cancer or cavities, they are all natural with no preservatives, artificial ingredients or pesticide residues. They are cholesterol free, naturally sweet, 100 per cent wholesome. And they are a completely renewable natural resource.

WHAT IS AFFECTING OUR HEALTH

Lets now go on a road of deduction outside of our body's jurisdiction as to what is affecting our health.

You may think I am being harsh and angry when you read the following. But in the interests of truth, I am prepared to say with passion, which may sound like anger, that I believe all Manufacturers be held responsible for their products **before** putting them on the supermarket shelves. Let the manufacturers be held accountable to know what additives such as colors/preservatives and food acids/flavors/bleaching agents/artificial sweetening/emulsifiers/ enzymes/flavor enhancers/flour treatment etc. affects the human body brain and mind.

Agents/humectants/propellants/thickeners/vegetable gums/compatibility of vitamins and minerals, etc., are still being used in preparations and food and do horrible things to the human brain /body/emotions and mind.

One of the most abominable things ever to happen to food is *irradiation*. There seems to be very little information to support use of this process on food that is supported by good scientific background. The idea of irradiation is for multinational food manufacturers to produce a longer shelf life for food after being irradiated by, as it seems, nuclear waste from nuclear power plants etc.

The following quotes are from the book **Food Irradiation The Facts by** Tony Webb and Dr Tim Lang of **THE LONDON FOOD COMMISSION,** an independent Body.

This book makes really interesting reading but make sure you eat first as you may be really upset at the mentality and heights some people's greed will take them to. The radiation on food, which as yet can't be detected, is at a rate 10 to 100 million times the dosage of a normal chest x-ray. What will it do to the workers working in the irradiation plants, especially if there is a radiation leak, or system malfunction? There is no instrumentation that can detect how many times the food has been irradiated at this time). Irradiation can inhibit sprouting of vegetables including potatoes, and delay ripening of fruits so they can be sent over longer distances. Meat products can have a shelf life of an almost indefinite period. The instruction for the preparation of meat for irradiation is really archaic. Dip the meat into sodium tripolyphosphate prior to irradiation. Tripolyphosphate is a chemical normally used for cleaning grime off walls as it cuts grease. This chemical is irritating to the skin and is used as a purgative.

A gigantic step backward for man. And they want us to eat this cardboard like dinosaur meat?

Irradiation kills microorganisms that lead to food spoiling such as yeasts, moulds, bacteria and reduce insect pests in grains such as wheat, rice or in spices. Irradiation can also be used to age spirits so will be of use to the brewing industry. Wine, whiskey and beers will be affected. Adverse affects have been observed in animals fed irradiated food and then the research papers were lost at a gigantic cost to taxpayers. Irradiation does severe damage to vitamins such as A, C, D, K, B2, B3, B6, B12 and Folic acid. Vitamin E is completely destroyed. Fruit juices suffer more from irradiation than the fungi it's meant to kill. Milk and milk products do not irradiate well as they hold the smell of radiation. Maybe too little is known about the massive and random rearrangements of the molecular structure of proteins, fats, carbohydrates, enzymes, and residual chemicals.

Conflicting evidence exists over whether or not irradiated food can cause mutation, genetic defects or chromosome defects in children. Enough, it's too depressing to think any one or any body of people could actually allow or think to allow this to go ahead. The people responsible cannot have any love for this planet, the people or the children yet to be born.

If this information is accurate then our immune systems are in for one hell of a tough time, and energetically it will be a miracle if we can cope. Maybe there is wisdom in booking a passage to the moon after all.

THE NEW ADDITIVE CODE BREAKER by Maurice Hanssen and Jill Marsden will also shock you as it explains the numbers written on packaging so then you can see what chemicals are put in the food.

Boycott food and drink that is not of the purest origin now and buy organic!
Your life and future generations depend on it!

Children's drinks and sweets have for years been full of flavors, additives and artificial colorings that have become like chemical cocktails of hyperactivity. My kids used to go wild and uncontrollable after drinking them. My partner and I used to hate our children going to other children's birthday parties unless we supervised them. Most times they would be so hyped up when they came back home, it would take a couple of hours to get them to settle down and get to bed.

Genetic Engineering

A gene from a cancer virus in chickens is implanted as a vector or carrier to implant a growth hormone into farmed fish so they will grow faster with no labelling stating this when sold.
A Brazil nut gene was inserted into soy and folks allergic to Brazil nuts were suddenly anaphylaxis, serious life threatening disease where one is not able to breathe.
The company responsible quickly removed the gene because the symptom was so dramatic.
Genes inserted into plants to make them resistant to certain pests, pesticides, herbicides, or antibiotics sound good, doesn't it?
Get the facts before you ingest this genetic modified untested or get proof of safety in this plague food.

Be responsible for what the children eat or be prepared to watch your kids suffer later with an immune problem. I hope not, but so many parents are not aware of the incredible damage done to children by saying they are young and can cope with it. Immune problems are starting younger and younger now as is seen by the younger cancer victims. Its only when we get older that the true damage comes out. It's too late then when you are at a funeral to say "sorry! I should have! I could have!" Its too late for them to see the cut flowers, your face pleading for forgiveness, when they lower the box in the gravesite! Its too late then, but not too late now to do something about your children or loved one's food!

Vaccinations

Before you put any foreign body in your or your child's system, please **be informed** as to what it is, where it came from, and what it is meant to do. Jock Doubleday is an expert on this subject and President of Natural man Natural woman, a non-profit organisation in California and can be e-mailed on jockdoubleday@aol.com

There are many homeopathic / herbal remedies which are accepted now and are so much better for your body and at no risk to your child or yourself.

If you have a reaction to any vaccine it could mean death or worse, so be aware.

Look the vaccine up on the Internet under the manufacturer and be informed!

Children have approximately 30 vaccination shots with side effects from meningitis to autism. Suggest you think before you give a vaccination to anyone check the facts. Joseph M. Mercola DO as reported in Townsend letter for doctors and patients writes that nobody really knows what toxic stews of chemicals and microorganisms we are having, and some authors are saying that aluminium and mercury is in every shot which could increase Alzheimer's in the future. Want to know more e-mail here dr@mercola.com)

Book Dr Viera Sceibner Ph.D on Vaccination 178 Govetts Leap Road Blackheath NSW 2785 Australia.

John Chamberlin

Foods and Additives

Having been brought up in a dysfunctional sibling family, I chose many life-threatening dis-eases in my life, as I wanted to leave the planet. I so foolishly thought this might be a way to leave the sorry and sad situations that I was co-creating and experiencing. I learnt that God, The Mother Father God, The Creator, The Universal Energy, Sumadhi, The Great Mysteries, or whatever else you would call the energies in charge of this Planet Earth, gave me free will. Because of that I had the free will to drink and eat anything I really wanted to and no ever one told me that there were food preservatives/flavors/additives in food like MONOSODIUM GLUTAMATE (621) which to my mind is a poison and affects the cerebral cortex nerves. It's meant to make food like meats taste better. Monosodium Glutamate was banned in the USA and now its back in full force again with different names. The last time I heard it was called hydrolysed plant protein and hydrolysed vegetable protein powder or enhancer). If you ever have Chinese food always ask that your food be cooked without monosodium if you are sensitive or you can expect a night of where you may not feel so well, or worse, 24 hours of sickness. It can give symptoms of tightening of the jaw muscles, numbness of the neck, chest and hands, thirst and nausea, palpitations, dizziness, fainting, pounding vice like headaches, and cold sweats.

You know, I foolishly expected everyone to do the right thing.
No one told me at a young age growing up on a farm that there was a thing called **greed** instead of **honor**.

I gave my power away expecting everyone to do the right thing. All the additives in food were poisoning me and other people without any lay people's knowledge.

Water And Filters

I believe in this day and age, it is our right to drink, bathe, and wash our vegetables and clothes in clean fresh water. Our bodies dictate we drink at least eight glasses a day for a healthy intestine and colon, and to pay for the disease ridden/parasite infested water that so many councils send to our homes laden with chlorine, is ridiculous. Yes, there is even parasite infestation in water among the chemicals, especially in some cities that recycle without adequate filters in their plants. I have seen and read documents which state chlorine is a derivative of aluminium that our immune systems cannot handle without great stress, sold a long time ago as a cockroach poison I believe.

We wonder why we get colds and are sick or often get unexplained rashes on our skin as our immune systems battle for supremacy against a lot of odds. There is even fluoride in our toothpaste and tests done by independent laboratories in Germany, Sweden and England state this was not good for our immune systems, so I guess someone else got paid as its now a choice in those countries. Besides, if it was so good for us why would companies that care about community health make so many millions of dollars manufacturing filters to filter it out. Filters for the whole house and shower are relatively inexpensive but imperative for good health.

Many swimming pools have been using chlorine and often there are people who have a low tolerance for it in their eyes and on their skin who end up with massive skin rashes, or extreme skin dryness. Chlorine is absorbed into the immune system through the skin, the largest organ of the body.

Using chlorine in a swimming pool is the old way to kill algae, bacteria, and viruses.

Why would you use chlorine in the pool when you can use a salt water chlorinator instead? Information can be obtained from Clearwater Products Australia Pty Ltd, PO Box 211 Glen Waverly Victoria 3150 Australia, Ph 03 9561-6577.on an instrument that produces its own chlorine gas when mildly salty water is passed through an electrolytic cell on the way to the pool. Salt is made up of two elements - sodium and chlorine. The chlorine gas dissolves instantly in the pool water, uses very little salt and goes to work to sanitize a pool immediately. Say goodbye to sore bloodshot eyes, strange colored hair, dry skin and rashes on the skin.

I have seen vegetables washed down in a supermarket showcase with Clorox bleach that is a poison to the human immune system but it does make vegetables look green and more desirable. Also a trick in some restaurants to get parsley to look good when it starts to droop is to put it in water with dish washing detergent then throw in the fridge for a few minutes, wash and serve. It may look good but what is that detergent on the parsley doing to our systems.

Learn for yourself about the fluoride risk and the evidence of a link to cancer by going to the following link. http://www.nofluoride.com

Bread

According to the American Federal Department Administration there is something like 150 chemicals in our bread by the time it is ready to eat, even bleach to make it white and a chemical that makes bread smell and taste like bread. Are we eating cardboard? Who would know?

Most people I know who are not well usually have their stomachs blow up with stomach gases after eating fresh bread. On testing clients with this problem and other dis-eases we find out that 90 per cent of these people have tested positive to wheat allergies. Approximately 50 per cent of the clients did not have the same test reactions when tested to organic wheat. This wheat had not been irradiated or sprayed on the farm to stop the weeds and bugs from growing to get a better crop.

Organic bread or Turkish bread is more expensive than ordinary bread, but well worth the difference when you get a good brand for your health. You can buy this bread at most Health Food shops and some modern supermarkets. Bread making machines using a top quality yeast from a health food store is also a good way to go. The wheat seed is sprayed to keep it from getting eaten before germination by bugs in the ground and again sprayed several times to keep the bugs and flies, butterflies, etc. and molds off the crop while growing. It is usually sprayed again once the crop is up, to keep the weeds at bay and subjected once more to stop weevils, bugs and mold when stored in storage bins. Preservative is added to the bread mixture to stop the moulds that are a rough form of penicillin, and again to assist with a long shelf life by preserving the bread. Yuk !

Soap

In our vanity to look great and attract a mate for our life experience we wash our bodies with trashy water and don't think about the chemicals or perfumes in the soap. We wonder why our skin is so dry and harsh and is so susceptible to rashes when under stress. A soap with tea-tree oil or aloe vera with out any other perfume does the job well as both tea tree oil and aloe vera are good for the skin. Shower filters are important to filter out the damaging toxins and chlorine. Cost approx $60.00 at WATER AND ICE shops in USA and most health shops in Australia.

Washing Powder

There are several doctors and researchers now saying that the chemicals in washing powders are responsible for the immune system weakness and it looks as though there will be some legislation coming soon to police this. A change to natural biodegradable washing powder is in order. For those who have very sensitive skin the fluid washing products seem to wash out of the clothes better than the powder cleansers. Sensitive area rashes usually get better with the change to liquid soap powders and by using a little less than recommended with lots of clear water rinses to wash the soap out. A friend told me once that he used a cold water cleanser and forgot to rinse his clothes twice and on going out in the rain he got into a lather. What was it doing to his skin rashes? Watch out for rashes if babies nappies and underclothes are not rinsed out properly too.

Hair shampoos and hair dyes

While they may give a great cosmetic appearance and be very effective, most shampoos and hair dyes will have some toxic ingredient which generally will react with our skin and bodies Aluminum again, among others. These are lathered into our hair to make us look glorious and feel great and hopefully get rid of any dandruff or dry skin. Half of the older organic hair shampoos used to make the hair too greasy and uncontrollable, but the newer brands are better.

Dare I mention HAIR DYES? All I ask is that you read and find out what the chemicals do to the human body and immune system, before you put them on your head again. For your health's sake, be aware of what you put on your head. With all the fine little veins and arteries so close to the skin surface of our heads and brains this is dangerous and if we continue these practices after being aware, we cannot complain or wonder why we have headaches or feel a lack of energy?

Sodium Laurel or Laureth Sulfate produces a lot of foam but is linked to cancer and is used to scrub garages floors and is strong. Squeaky-clean hair huh? It is difficult to find a shampoo and conditioner without it but if you cannot then go to your local health store and the proprietors will be happy to oblige you. Now days the organic products are much more efficient and nice to use and I am sure the animals will thank you if it is not tested for efficiency on animals too!

To be forewarned is to be forearmed.

Perfumes

I love to smell a good perfume, but most perfumes today are good chemicals and to get the best out of the chemicals they are designed to sink into the skin and are usually applied on the veins of the wrist or a cotton ball between the breasts. All are designed to enter the skin so when applied to warm skin with veins close to the surface, incredibly as it seems your perfume could be slowing you and your energy up if you have allergies to what is in it.

Even today we have perfume and after shave you girls and guys should be aware of. This perfume/after shave comes complete with pheromones in them that will increase and attract the sex drive of a perfect stranger within nose range of the aromas. There are many naturally scented oils that can be a good alternative and won't affect your skin or your immune system.

Make-up

Be very careful when choosing your type of make up as most of the skin complaints for the face have been caused by inferior make-up products. There are many good natural products on the market now that does not use animal testing to test the product. www.biopacificskincare.com.au.
Bio-pacific skincare 07-3205-3055 in Australia.

Toothpaste

Any toothpaste with sodium laureth sulfate in it to cause bubbles may be in your best interest to avoid as that beauty has links to cancer too. Organic is best. www.o-n-e.com.au for genesis certified organic toothpaste or see your local naturopath.

Deodorants

Most underarm deodorants contain aluminum, preservatives and perfumes, and when applied have almost direct contact with the veins and lymphatics under the arms and breast and feeds into the immune system. Excess aluminum has been linked to the disease of Alzeimers, dis-ease and Dementia.

Anti-perspirants prevent you from perspiring, thereby inhibiting the body from purging toxins from below the armpits and as these toxins do not magically disappear they are lodged or deposited in the lymph nodes below the arms or beside or under the breast since the body cannot sweat it out.

Nearly all breast cancers / tumors occur in the upper outside quadrant of the breast area which is precisely where the lymph nodes are located. Men are less likely to be affected as some of the anti-persperant is caught up in the hair. Don't use this if you have just shaved under the arms, as the chemicals will enter through the fine cuts.

Heavy bags draped over the shoulder misdirect/dam up the blood and lymph and can trap it under the arm in the lymph nodes too.

Aluminium pots pans, saucepans, pop drinks, beer cans, etc.

Cooking in aluminium pots is really asking for trouble, as when they get hot and cool down the pots will leave a residue of aluminium. If the cook is like me and burns food occasionally then invariably scrapes the pot when taking produce out some aluminium gets in the food.

When used to get burnt food off, pot scrubbers leave residues of aluminum which is readily consumed in our ignorance as the filings are so fine and hard to see with the naked eye.

High levels of aluminum have been found in Alziemer's and dementia patients. Aluminum can be taken out of the system by doing a heavy metal detoxification with herbs. See your naturopath or write to Helen Kroeger Herbs 1122 Pearl St. Boulder Colorado 80302 or www.herbalhealer.com for de-toxing Herbal extracts.

It is so easy to purchase Pyrex glass pots, pans and even fry pans at inexpensive prices. Stainless steel pots and pans are also good after a good wash out, although they are a lot more expensive.

Soft drinks, pop, beer sold in aluminum cans or steel should be avoided in my opinion for much the same reason. Many times on tipping out the drink and looking at what is left in it in the sun reflection, I have been able to see little glistening fibers of aluminum reflecting happily away at me. Try it for yourself, but know that some cans are better than others for seeing this.

Do you know that checking food for vitality on the SE-5 Intrinsic Data Field Analyzer before putting in the oven to cook can show normal high vitality? The SE-5 measures subtle energies.

In a control experiment a potato was cut in half and one piece wrapped in aluminum foil. The two pieces were cooked alongside each other and the foiled half tested with no vitality at all at the finish of cooking. The other piece of potato did not drop much in vitality at all.

Multinational companies who make billions of dollars selling aluminum will defend their product at all costs as they have nothing to lose and a lot to gain, as I have already found out on a radio show in Perth Australia, when I spoke about avoiding aluminum residue in the body.

Please do not take my word for it, make your own inquiries and talk to your friendly local naturopath, homeopathic doctor or do some tests for yourself. Make a stand for your health by using and buying products in glass that can be recycled again and again and help to save our environment. There is a place for aluminum, but not in our food, drinks, or in products we put on our bodies.

The following report No 540 by McGugan for the Federal Trade commission of the U.S. Government Washington DC advises that the sale of aluminum wares for cooking is prohibited in Germany, Great Britain, Brazil, France, Switzerland, Belgium, Hungary, and Austria.
Also that cooking in Aluminum can cause the following.
Boiling water in aluminum produces hydro-oxide poison
Boiling eggs in aluminum produces phosphate poisoning
Boiling meat in aluminum produces chloride poisoning
Cooking bacon in aluminum produces powerful narcotic that can cause an individual to slip into coma or death.
Boiling soda in aluminum produces hydro-oxide of sodium
Vegetables cooked in aluminum are made poisonous by the production of hydro-oxide
Aluminum produces a drug that neutralizes the digestive juices of the stomach, robbing them of their value to digest food and causing or producing stomach ulcers and colitis.
The poison produced by aluminum brings about a condition of acidosis of the blood. This condition destroys the red blood cells which produces a condition similar to anaemia.

For cooking safely
Use ironware, stainless steel, granite or porcelain coated, or glass such as Pyrex

Alcoholic Drinks

Alcoholic drink is really loved by most of us, and even taken to excess by some of us on the odd occasion. Me too, in moderation. Some wines tested are full of weed and pesticide residue.

Oils are sprayed on grapevines to keep the weed killer and bug killer on the plant during the heavy rains. Excess oils are impossible to soak or wash off the grapes in the vats and so the taste and residue of weed and pesticides is still there in the finished product. There have been many itinerant Mexican workers die a horrible death from poisoning because they were hungry and didn't wash grapes before eating them. Sulfides and quickeners are added to make the wines more palatable so they can be sold more quickly. Remember also the preservative used to stop this conglomeration from going off, to give longer shelf life, to cut losses and to prevent the product from being sent back. Ever have spots of skin on your tongue just disappear? It's usually rather sore for a couple of days until it grows back. Now you know what causes it. Maybe the brew is only a couple of months old and in days gone past would not have been sold under 4-5 years without the chemicals.

Why is it that men and woman who enjoy their beer are getting fatter and fatter with huge beer bellies? I believe alcohol, energetically speaking, has little to do with why most people get so sick from excess drinking the next day although it would contribute to it. Our immune systems are not being able to cope and excrete all the chemicals, preservatives and additives used to make the drink taste appealing. If all this is happening, we are drinking a Molotov cocktail for our immune systems. Being overloaded, our natural filters are not able to protect our brain functions from excess dangerous chemicals and toxicity, and therefore we become lethargic and tired as our bodies try to cope in overload.

While I don't think that alcoholic drinks are good for our immune systems, I do believe we are meant to experience life on this planet and have been shown that everything in moderation is OK. Don't complain if you cannot remember anything after a night of excess

drinking.   Alcohol dries up or uses all the Vitamin B and C in our bodies and brain.
An excess of alcohol and drugs can and will destroy memory cells.

TIP. Massive doses of vitamins B and C can sometimes alleviate a hangover but leave at least 10 minutes between taking each one of them as they do not mix energetically.

If you decide to give up alcoholic drinks and wish to regenerate your memory, pure Royal Jelly at dosage rates of at least 1000mg in capsule form to be taken at least twice a day has been known to regenerate brain cells. Capsules, with no extras or additives. PURE if you can get it.
Do not purchase Royal Jelly in honey drink vials from well-meaning health shop proprietors.
Royal Jelly is expensive but highly recommended. This worked for me after totally losing my memory after having a minor heart attack from a combination of an overdose of medically given morphine and years of drinking alcohol and stress. It took more than two years of gradual retention until now my memory is restored. I am able to stand and give seminars all weekend now without looking at notes.

An added benefit for the men is that Royal Jelly can also help with premature ejaculation too.
Research has shown that our bodies can totally regenerate in every seven to eight years for all cells except our memory cells. We have a totally new body in seven to eight years, so start now. Whatever age you are, it's never too late to start to regenerate. Recycle your body and brain now.

Milk and Dairy Products

Let's look at milk. MOTHER'S MILK is good for us as it gives us all the antibiotics to survive in the colostrum. However, cow's milk is not the same unless it is straight from the cow. How can any product still be good for us when it comes from the cow, and by the time it is pasteurized, homogenized, added vitamins etc., takes

so many days to get to us. If the milk butterfat is too high, it was watered down from the tap water to the required butterfat. With too much butterfat there was too much cream on top and so it was harder to wash out the bottles, with the bottles and cartons smelling more of milk going off. Besides, you can sell more cream if the milk doesn't have a little floating on top. If we want cream, milk companies can separate this to get more money, or water it down and get paid for unfiltered water
I had the opportunity to work in a milk factory once and have not found the need to drink milk much since.

Do you know that the major test to find out how much radiation is in the atmosphere uses milk?
Milk holds radiation easily and the powers that be wish to irradiate the milk. Scary huh?

Having milked cows as a youth and a man growing up, it was common knowledge that a sick cow's milk was put in the holding vats if the quota was a little short, but it was strained to make sure the mastitis didn't show up. The milk was treated at the factory, right? Pasteurized, sterilized etc. It was irresponsible and everyone who were milking cows did it on the quiet and it was done in ignorance, as farmers didn't know any better at the time. Penicillin, oreomysin, hormones and other concoctions were put in the udder in the cow's body to stop infection, stop lumpy diseased milk, and make a sick cow well. This milk was not meant to be sold but saved to give to the calves or the dogs to drink, or be thrown out.

You can't blame the farmer as half the time he or she was just trying to survive and did it in ignorance thinking the factory would take care of it. Penicillin and a lot of antibiotics now don't work on a lot of people as they have allergic reactions to it, maybe an unknowing overdose of it from milk and meat.

There is even a hormone developed to make the cow produce more milk. This has not been tested enough and could be damaging to the human immune system. What about the hormones that are fed to the beef cows and steers to make them grow fast so the producer can sell them quicker. Ever wondered what effect this has to our bodies and to why our kids are so overweight and are getting so big? It used to be that children with few exceptions used to grow to within 6 inches of their parents' height and size. Not any more. Buy organic milk and meat and enjoy the taste we used to have when we were younger. If you drink milk and have a sore or bloated stomach within the next half-hour you could be lactose intolerant so a test will be necessary.

It appears strange but it seems that our bodies can go into a self punishment at times and crave foods that react to us the most.

Soy

I had the misfortune to miss drinking milk because of allergic reactions and had not found an organic supplier. I decided to accept the advertising blurb that soy was the bee's knees and good for you too. WRONG!

My cappaccinos were delicious but I got stiffer and more swollen in the joints until I realised what it was that was causing my rapid bringing on of the Old man syndrome, and thought I would have to give up work, and I was not able to afford that. My hands and joints in my body just ached and burned like a fire going on inside. I did some research and got scared with what I read on soy, and stopped immediately and started detoxing. It still took several months of taking supplements of Lanes shark cartilage, Glucosamine sulfate and Natural Salmon fish oil or Flax oil internally and Emu oil topically on the affected joints for the pain to leave my hands. Its back to organic milk or filtered water for me now.   www.mercola. com/feb13/more_on_soy.htm

Too Good to be True and www.soyonlineservice.co.nz)

There are many young children who can have allergies to milk and soy in formulas so be aware!

Chickens and laying hens are given hormones and additives in their food to keep them from getting disease from being cooped up in very inhumane situations. Organic free range fed chickens and eggs for me and even then there is no guarantee that these chickens are not feeding on weed sprayed pasture.

Pork is no better if you see all the trash that most people give these scavengers. They will eat anything, and if it is not overcooked it is possible to get a disease called trichinosis and other weird and wonderful worm and parasite infested diseases. If you must eat it have it cooked really well and remember the apple as this does have an affect of reducing the toxicity and of cancelling out the worms. In some poor overseas countries, I have been told that it is hard to tell the difference between human flesh and pork, so pork is not for me anymore unless I know where it comes from.

Fish is wonderful when fresh, unless irradiated, fished out of polluted water, or stored too long and becomes stale and hard because of marketing strategies. Like fish, eggs can be left too long in so-called market cooperatives in efforts to hold the prices high and not flood the markets.
For great taste buy fresh and organic.

No I am not vegetarian anymore but I am discriminating as to the freshness of what I eat, and where it comes from! If it comes from a third World country be really careful.
Rat, cat, dog, or horse can be served with beautiful flavors that will palate please.

I have known several clients who used to only purchase Asian food stuffs and as our immune systems are not brought up to cope with these strange bugs from foreign states, became very sick and it took them a long time to isolate what it was and where the bug came from. We also need to know that the cleanliness in some countries is not to the standard our bodies are used too.
Be discriminating and support your local grower, manufacturers wherever possible as the energies of where you live will be better for your body anyway as nature has a wonderful way of providing missing and balancing energies when eating locally.

I had a friend once who worked for a delicatessen and small goods wholesaler. He told me that if someone wanted bacon rashes and the company he worked for didn't have any, he was required to make up some from mutton, lamb or second grade meat using chemicals to make it taste and smell the same. By charging a lot less for it, it was not questioned and he defied his friends to tell the difference. Be aware. It's a chemical world.

If you have had enough, turn to the next chapter where we cover how we can alleviate these problems. I am not asking you to believe everything and anything you are told, but please question all foods and liquids you put in your body for fuel! You won't put petrol in a fire knowingly will you, but some of the additives to food could do the same damage to your insides by us not being aware.

Know that our bodies are intricate machines of whirling energies that can cope with massive amounts of abuse of eating harmful foods and drinks for a long time, and cope with amazing stressful situations and still keep going. If we are not aware enough to avoid the GARBAGE IN GARBAGE OUT theory it will eventually catch up with us, and we will feel dreadful and want to die because there is no joy or quality of life. We have no one to blame but ourselves by continuing to expect everyone else to do the right thing. It's too late for that. The crisis is here now!

Vitamin /Minerals

Even though there are many vitamin/mineral manufacturers who are working really hard to be honest and ethical companies, there are also companies who capitalize on greed and are out for the quick buck. They make it their business to sell vitamins and minerals at a cheaper price than most do on the market or in their greed cheat.

While some high integrity, motivated, dedicated people are doing their best to give good value they find they are competing with the rip-off merchants. Many of these products are being checked by researchers like Dr See who before he joined Mannatech Incorporated worked on a grant from the National Institute of Health in UC Irvine

California and found many vitamins /minerals /herbal products / supplements were out of integrity. Some 90 per cent of over 450 products tested were either toxic or a placebo and the vast majority had enormous variations from what was printed on the label. Some vitamin C was literally void of a vitamin C and products whose actual content was 10 times what was printed on the label.

The Mannatech product of Ambrotose, a glyconutritional dietary supplement, is a great product with good results but is very expensive and is sold similar to a pyramid selling scheme.

 The vitality of the body electric's matching with a lot of vitamins and minerals by checking with various instruments has found a lot of preparations to have less integrity than that of sawdust or cardboard. The irradiated varieties are not for me to recommend either, thank you. I read recently on the Internet how some researchers were saying that garlic was no good as it was full of radiation. On tracking down where it came from, it was found the garlic had been irradiated and so common sense says that as garlic absorbs free radicals /toxins /irradiation in our bodies, then it would if irradiated absorb as much radiation as it could. Duh!

Get a naturopath to teach you how to test your body with kinesiology and teach you about the compatibility of the vitamins/ minerals you are buying for your body and to suggest what products and brands are the best for you.

Know that some brands do not mesh with your body although they may be good for other members of your family.

Diets

A diet will not do much for you unless you really believe it. There are so many get rich quick merchants throwing diets on the market that every time you turn around there is another one. Sometimes these are another version of a diet that was banned a few years ago. None of them will be any good for you unless you believe it will.

Remember, this is a billion dollar industry and having the desperate emotive desire to make it work can sometimes make it work, hopefully for a long time without too much effort in starvation or denial. Remember that most times the person selling it to you is motivated to be thin, trim and to make money by selling it to others. It's in your best interest to check out the motivation of these people, wade through the sales pitch and get to the nitty gritty.

To my mind nothing will substitute for good healthy balanced eating and a guide suggested by your naturopath or someone who understands the balance of foods.

A certified hypnotherapist will help you find out the cause of why you are self-punishing yourself and what trauma started this program of excess weight. Reprogramming the subconscious mind to take the time to eat healthy food in a balanced, quiet, stress-free environment is really important.
Quite often it can be a simple program from childhood where the stressed parent not knowing how to comfort a crying child stuffs food into it mouth to shut it up, just in case it is hungry.
This translates into whenever I am stressed /depressed or not feeling well, I need to stuff myself with food.

Macrobiotics is a good method to look into and learn. This method aims to promote longevity principally by diet consisting chiefly of whole grains, vegetables, fish and other natural foods. Convection ovens, wok cooking using less fat are a good investment in health. Avoid fatty dressings on salads flavor enhancers etc. Raw fresh organic food and some vegies and fruit juices will do more for you than all the expensive diets.
If you do not have the time then the Biotta brand juices are 100 per cent pure and natural organic and taste beautiful.
Address for Biotta AG. CH-8274 Tagerwilen Switzerland but you should find them in your health store.

Find a SE-5 Intrinsic Data Field Analyzer operator or a Vegatest Expert 752 test or similar to establish what foods you have allergies to, have them balanced, then avoid the foods to which you have low tolerance. In this way we can stop the self-punishment cycle the body will sometimes put us through by craving and eating foods that will repeat on us.

Environment

Have you ever looked at where you live in a critical way? Environmental pollution is here to stay in a big way, and the more sensitive we are the worse it is for us. Buy or borrow a sensitive car radar sensor and drive round your home noticing how many times its bells and whistles go off as it picks up microwave activity.

There is an incredible level of telecommunication microwaves, TV communication, computers, power line leakage, mobile telephones, aircraft radar landing beams and signals, motion sensor lights and burglar and fire alarms operating which can all together or singularly affect our health.

I had a personal experience of a young child standing close in front of a TV and fell to the ground just as a plane flew overhead which the mother remembered later and informed me.

The little girl was admitted to hospital and the doctor said that it looked as if all her brain circuits were not working. We tracked a airport radar landing beam that went right over the house and must have been switched on precisely when the little girl stood in front of a blurry reception, trying to see what was on the screen. Thank God she is OK now but took many years for her to recover as an epileptic.

In some men's urinals special waves are emitted at stomach level to flush the urinal when one moves away. You can check your house using a gauss meter to measure the low frequency waves emitted in your house. It's sometimes amazing what's in your house that can be out of balance or coming from a leaky transmitter or sub station near by
.

Humanity now has no choice and putting one's head in the sand like the ostrich, hoping it will go away or get better, will not help. We will need to adapt our bodies to these waves as no governing body is likely to ever have the intestinal fortitude nor the manpower to stop and test the effects these waves and instruments have on our systems. Be aware and avoid the waves where possible. Skip the public urinal and wait until you get home or find a lonely tree.

Pollutants in Home and Automobile

Many people have experienced up to six to twelve months some problems listed here from new homes or vehicles. Sometimes by opening the whole new place up for a month or so before moving in the irritations were reduced.

Some of the sources and symptoms are:

Benzene, paint, new carpets, upholstery - headaches, eye/skin irritation, fatigue, cancer

Ammonia, tobacco smoke, cleaning supplies - eye/skin irritation, headaches, nose bleeds, sinus problems.

Chloroform, paint, new drapes, upholstery, new carpeting - headaches, asthma, attacks, dizziness, eye irritation, skin irritation.

Formaldehyde, tobacco smoke, plywood, cabinets, furniture, particle board, office dividers, new carpets, new drapes, wallpaper panelling - headaches, eye/skin irritation, drowsiness, fatigue, respiratory problems, memory loss, depression, gynaecological problems, cancer.

Benzopyrene, tobacco smoke - asthma attacks, eye/skin irritation, sinus problems, lung cancer.

Hydrocarbons, tobacco smoke, gas burners, furnaces - headaches, fatigue, nausea, dizziness, breathing difficulty.

Trichlorethylene, paints, glues, furniture, wallpaper - headaches, eye/skin irritations, respiratory irritation.

Xylene, paint, new carpets, cleaning supplies - headaches, dizziness, fatigue

Paint

Some forms of plastic paint will give off noxious fumes and can make a person very sick so it is best to leave or sleep in another room for a week or so until the fumes dissipate.

Carpet glues

Carpet glues are also able to give off chemicals that last for a very long time within the home or office environment.

Wallboards

Like some chipboards have been known to contain a chemical that caused a child to get bad asthma which left her when they moved house.

Then we have things like dust mites, bacteria, dust, pollens, bacteria, mosquitos, midges no see ums, sand flies, etc which can also play havoc with our allergies. Over 40 per cent of the population are believed to have allergies of some sort or another. The Allergy Bible by Linda Gamlin gives a great insight into understanding and treating allergies and intolerances

TV & Radio

Don't let you or your children fall asleep in front of the TV or radio, as even though it's been outlawed in The United States, subliminal programming still occurs to get you to buy special products. I got caught once watching a certain graphic ad for a cold medicine and started to get sick immediately after. These messages are either too low or high for the human ear, too quick for the human eye, but are picked up and recorded by the subconscious mind to get you to buy a certain product. A TV of mine went out of balance at one time and I was amazed at what was written on the screen. Negative news and videos designed to scare will negatively program the subconscious mind into deep hidden fear. More stories on uncontrollable fears caused by this programming later. Do you know that a hypnosis disc running in a circular motion in really bright colors is being used in advertisements and on the can of a new brand of soft drink in

Australia? This drink is selling really well and the local authorities are doing nothing about it at this time.

Electricity Lines

Living close to electrical transformers or overhead power lines and mobile phone boosters /transmitters can also be hazardous to your health. There have been many cases of leukemia, immune system problems in people living too close to a leaky transformer. Maybe that what's wrong with me? I used to live under several high-tension wires for several years and on a damp, drizzly or foggy day, our hair would stand on end as we drove the tractor under it. The milking shed was close to it and the cows would kick like hell as they got minor electric shocks from the milking cups put on their teats and udders to take the milk.

Remember that our bodies are made up of millions of electrical circuits and are very delicate. Purchase a gauss meter or talk to your local authorities.

Mobile Phones Computer Screens

Electromagnetic radiation is linked to cancer so prevention is always better than cure.

Radiation differs from phone to phone and exposure up to three milligauss per hour is regarded to be safe. The safest way is to not use them but if your need to communicate is great then get an earplug to the phone to get away from the radiation. Remember not to leave the mobile on your hip too long if you are talking for a long time if you wish to have mobility in the future.

I have seen people with massive headaches and cancer in the ears caused by irritation/radiation from mobile phones. The court cases of the future will be just like the tobacco industry.

Computer screens can be bought to cut down radiation and reduce eyestrain, but remember to ground the screen as instructed. Many people have reported after fitting these that they do not get the tension headaches, are not so tired, less stiff, and they still have their eyesight at the end of the day.

Underground streams

Water streams running under where we sleep can cause a negative electromagnetic field in your home. A skilled practitioner, a dowser using copper wire and rods to re-route the negative, disruptive fields can easily change these disruptive streams such as Geopathic Stress lines, Hartmann lines, etc. There are real dangers of sleeping on a Hartmann line and if your bedroom or work areas lie over these lines which are six to eight feet apart depending where you live there is a good chance for a serious health problem. Dr Ernst Hartmann has 40 years of documentation to back this up and states that for optimal health a person needs to sleep in a neutral Hartmann zone. He has discovered that the lines appear as a grid and cover the whole earth similar to the aura of the earth. He states that if you sleep on a north /south line you are prone to cramps and rheumatism and on an east /west line you are prone to inflammations. Babies placed in a crib on a Hartmann line will cry like mad and if you move the crib off the line it will stop crying. Where the Hartmann lines cross if over your bed or work place there is a good chance for major disease like cancer and heart disease. www.earthtransitions.com/sleeping. htm for more information or E-mail EarthHeal99@aol.com for a practitioner near you.

Feng Shui

This is an ancient art used by the Chinese for centuries for balance and harmony in the home and I have heard seen and felt incredible changes once the home has been Feng Shui. Much is written about energies, environmental harmony and books on the subject are easily obtainable form your local bookstore and can be easily understood with practice or a small class in it.

Spraying our pests and bugs

The bugs that invade our homes being sprayed is fine for those who like to do that. However, there are safer and more humane ways now available than spraying a mild nerve gas or one that uses similar principles on them. Have you ever seen the agonizing death these cause?

While it's OK to spray or mist the carpet or accessible areas, it's not OK to allow a baby or pets to crawl or play on the same carpet. Parents, please put a sheet down before baby goes on the floor if you must spray.

We may wonder why we feel so queasy after walking barefoot through an area we sprayed. Your veins and arteries are really close to the surface on your feet, hands, head and genitals if you sit down. A friend who walked barefoot then sat on the carpet to read some papers, got extremely sick shortly after and ended up in hospital emergency. There is a ward in a Gold Coast hospital which nurses call the Baygon ward after all the people who did not take precautions. There are several low cost alternatives that don't make people and pets sick.

Cigarettes Tobacco and Marijuana

Then we have cigarettes. I can hear you say, Oh God now this, especially if you are a cigarette smoker, but surprise! It is better for you to smoke a few cigarettes a day than take heavy drugs to keep you calm if you are a nervous person. However, be careful. An acquaintance had a heart attack while smoking. After finding the normal preservatives in the tobacco but not finding the cause of the attack, the hospital found the paper around the tobacco had traces of an irritant chemical to get the smoker to smoke more. Is this why there is so much lung cancer? In days gone by people could smoke and basically stay in good health living to a ripe old age. There is refrigerated, guaranteed weedicide and pesticide free, organic tobacco now being sold in the USA. For those of you who cannot give it up, that's your choice, but please don't smoke around others like me. Many of us were exposed to that as children and we have no tolerance for smoke, have allergies to cigarette smoke and get sinus blockages immediately. Smoking around food is dangerous and plainly shows a lack of respect for anyone, including yourself. A secondary smoker is more at risk of getting cancer than the person smoking gets.

What is in cigarette smoke?

Information gathered from the Board of Health Collaborative Cape Cod regional Tobacco control program in The United States.

Butane - cigarette lighter fluid
Carbon monoxide - car exhaust fumes
Methanol - rocket fuel
Methane - swamp gas
Arsenic - poison
Ammonia - floor / toilet cleaner
Cadmium - rechargeable batteries
Ethanol - alcohol
Acetone - nail polish remover
Hexamine - barbecue lighter
Formaldehyde - preserves body tissue & fabric
DDT/Dieldrin - insecticides
Acetic acid - vinegar
Hydrogen cyanide - gas chamber poison
Naphthalene - moth balls
Over 4000 chemicals - Over 43 cancer causing agents

An experiment was carried out at a Californian university where approximately one hundred students were offered $100 if they could recognize their own brand of cigarette. Twenty tubes from various brands of cigarette were set up, for the students to smoke to identify their regular brand. What the organizers didn't tell them was that five of the tubes had hot air coming through them. Only one person picked his brand and most chose the hot air ones as being their brand.

Another thing to know is that from Indian Yogi books on breathing, a smoker is really doing the relaxation breath. This is to sit upright and draw the breath in imagining a white light from your scource filling your lungs, then hold the breath for at least five seconds. Breathe out slowly and longer in the out breath and hold the breath for five seconds on the complete exhalation. This is to be continued for at least five minutes for maximum benefit. And fresh air is free.

It is seen in the aura that in smoking marijuana a crack opens up on the etheric/astral levels and you leave yourself open to all sorts of weird and wonderful astral earthbound souls. It's amazing to find that marijuana gives the smoker the effects of being really intelligent and carrying on an intelligent conversation. I have news for those smokers, please tape yourself on a tape recorder, and play back a couple of days after the experience. Most listeners or practitioners who are not partaking usually have to wait for long periods of time for a marijuana smoker to say anything intelligent and this becomes very boring for the listener during the short circuit wait periods.

A long-term marijuana user comes out with very beautiful blue eyes, but a naturopath who knows will tell you it's because the brain does a short-circuit and the organs and body imperfections are not registered in the eye.. Most therapists will not work on anyone in this mind state, as their minds are too unstable because they drift away too much for any accuracy. Reference is from the book Science of Iridology.

The Medical Journal of Australia Vol 156 April 6, 1992 is good unbiased reading and my interpretation if you are a marijuana smoker is this. How are you going to be able to explain to your kids why they are not able to have children because you liked smoking the substance.

This is minor compared to the fetotoxicity, cancer, and impairment of psychomotor performance, schizophrenia, long term impairment of memory to say the least. The dealers want to grow and sell as quickly as possible without being caught by the police department so have a guess at what weedicide pesticide and herbicides you think you are smoking. Russian roulette would be safer.

The Medical Journal of Australia April 6th, 1992 states that marijuana or hashish, which is from the cannabis plant and produces symptoms of neuro behavioural toxicity, disrupts all phases of gonadal or reproductive function, and is fetotoxic. Does this mean that nature does not want to reproduce those who desecrate the body brain and mind and make weaker strains of human?

Long-term memory loss is prevalent in adolescents, prolonged impairment of psychomotor performance, a sixfold increase in the incidence of schizophrenia, cancer of the mouth, jaw, tongue, and lungs in 19 to 30 year olds. Fetotoxicity and non-lymphobiastic leukemia in children of a marijuana-smoking mother are only some of the problems. Why in the world would you want to do that to yourself and your family? You must be missing a few cogs in the wheel of life if you are looking for good health and continue with this inconsiderate behaviour which not only affects your health and the health of your children.

Your children will be really angry with you if they find out they cannot reproduce because of your habit. Look at your self-image, and think about why you don't want to be here on this planet with us and start to create a better place here for the future generations.

AND WE BLAME GOD FOR OUR MISERABLE WEAK EXISTENCE OF A NON JOY, NON FULFILLED LIFE.

God gave us choice, so you have the choice now to make the changes to your life that needs to be challenged /changed and be aware, for it is not going to be or get any better without all of us humans making an effort. Our bodies are wonderful pieces of energy and can cope with a lot of stress and garbage that we put into our systems. I am not against anyone making a living and feel directors of companies, not the government, need to be more responsible, and as the buyer of healthy products, we must be more aware and educated to know what we put into our bodies.

Claim our power back, and vote with our feet and our checkbook. Buy balanced products, wholesome food and the appropriate cleansers we need to nourish and adorn our bodies.

Leave products and companies that don't care about the general public to their own demise.

It's time to demand rights to good health, good nourishing food and pure water which is our birthright!

THE BODY, CONSCIOUS, SUBCONSCIOUS MIND AND EMOTIONS ARE ALL ENERGY IN MOTION

Let's start at the beginning.

For us to understand how to heal ourselves, the whole body, mind and emotions, is a moving mass of energy kept together by our souls. The science of Kirlian photography shows very fine energy lines that show up in high frequency photography.

In other words, if you take a neutron microscope and could look at your hand through the microscope, you would find your hand a whole moving mass of meshing atomic particles called neutrons, electrons, etc., particles going round and round in circles and cycles. When our souls leave or die for any reason, our bodies disintegrate, fall apart and go back to dust.

The aura that clairvoyants see is the energy that swirls around the body and when there is a pain, imbalance, or problems of imbalance, this shows up in the aura as a dark spot, a grayish area or sometimes red flashes. This all indicates unbalanced energy to the person who is looking. Different clairvoyants see different colors depending on how they were taught to perceive them.

When someone is on my table or I am teaching in my seminar on Self-Healing we feel these imbalances. The energies can be hot, cold, or fluctuating depending on the density. The so-called thickness of this energy indicates the severity of the pain or imbalance, and usually each person has a slightly different frame of reference.

This energy is around all living things. On a following page you will see photos taken by a brilliant man called Grayden Rixton who is one of the pioneers in this field. These photos show a hand with the energy coming off it as it rests on the camera film. If a person is taught how to read these prints and is skilled enough he will tell what energy circuits in your body are in or out of balance. Generally speaking the absence of energy will reflect what organ is out of balance, similar to Acupuncture meridian charts.

Acupuncture /Acupressure/Meridians

The Chinese have for centuries told us about energies and meridians which are the main trunk lines of energy running through our bodies. They have been operating on this energy system using fine acupuncture needles for the purpose of re-establishing or balancing energy flows through meridians of the body, to stimulate energy to specific organs or energy centers to bring about change for the positive. Acupressure also triggers these energy points but to a lesser degree. However, this practice can be learnt in a much shorter time than acupuncture and there are several books on this. The first set of illustrations show the meridians or main energy circuits going through the body and ending at the fingers, toes, ears and eyes.

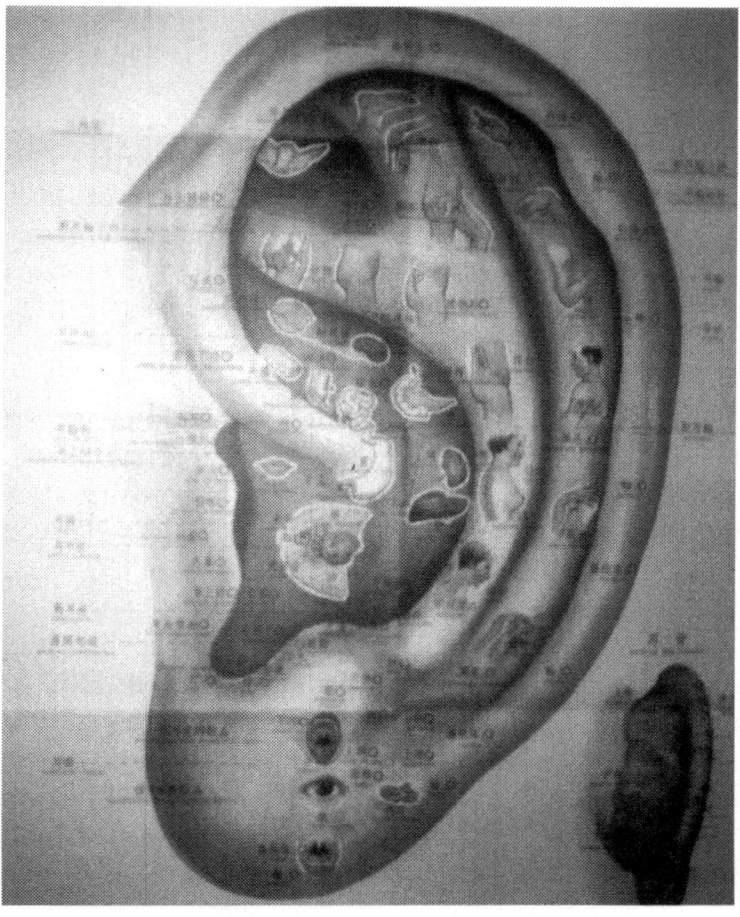

The following hands and feet depict approximate organ points in Reflexology so get massaging.

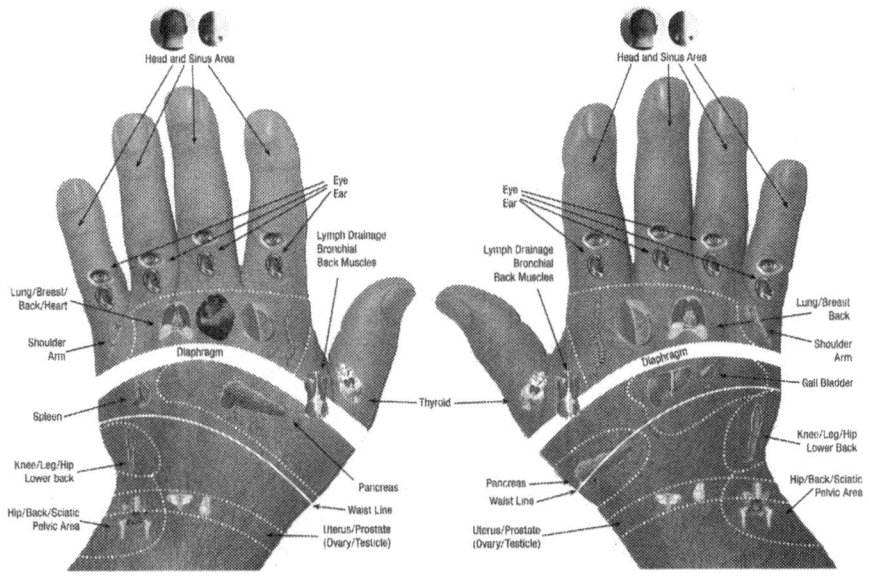

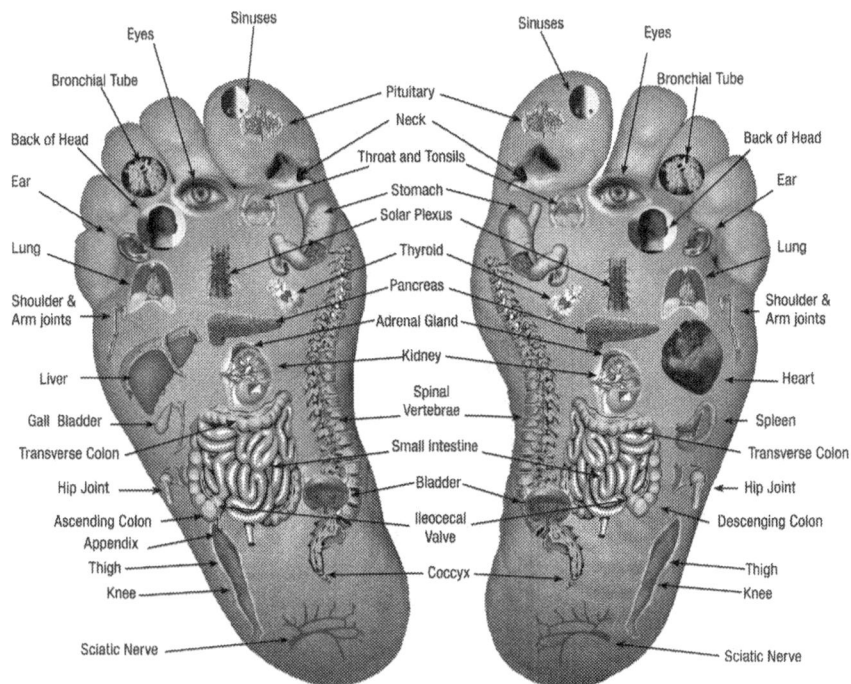

Meridians

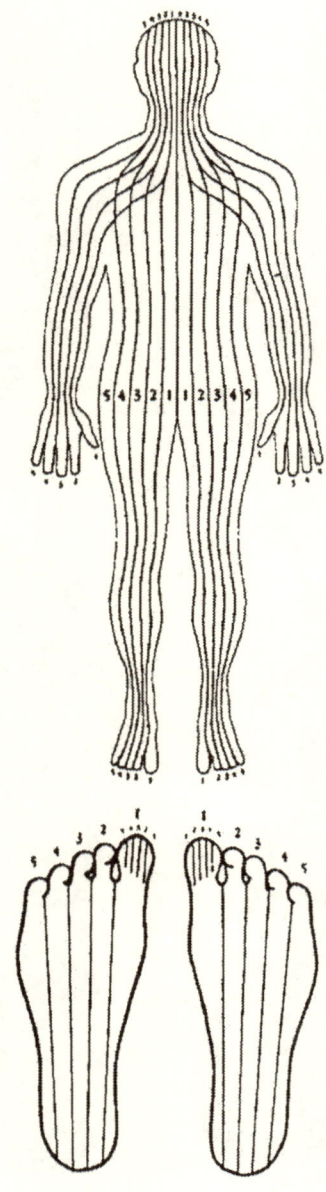

Iridology

This is the science and study of the eye whereby the iris tissue of the eye reflects physical and psychological patterns of the individual giving the ability to understand how he will react to the environment and it reveals the bodies strengths and weaknesses, emotional reactivates, communication and learning modes. Or simpler put, where all your road maps can be read and it doesn't have to be in the morning after the night out on the town either.

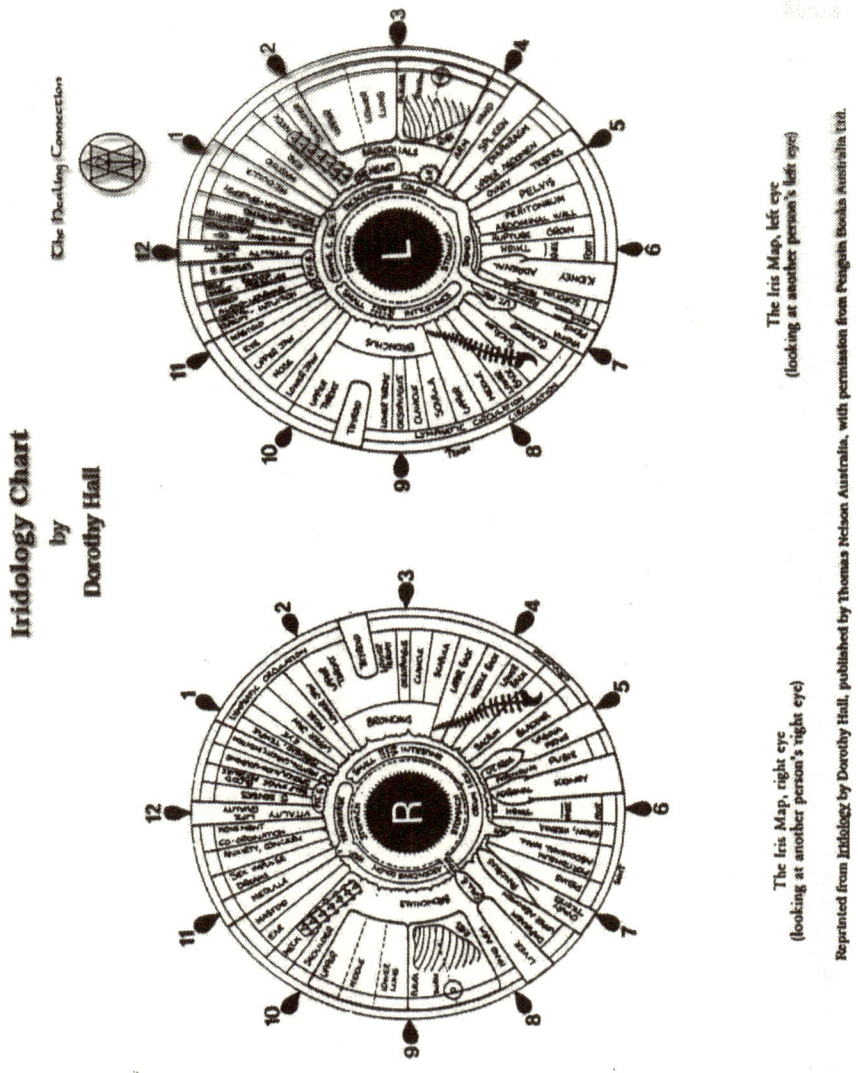

Iridology Chart
by
Dorothy Hall

The Iris Map, left eye
(looking at another person's left eye)

The Iris Map, right eye
(looking at another person's right eye)

Reprinted from Iridology by Dorothy Hall, published by Thomas Nelson Australia, with permission from Penguin Books Australia Ltd.

I suggest you buy a book on Iridology by Dorothy Hall and learn this or take a course in it, as you can with practice know where you are having problems or short circuits within your body.

It is really surprising what the eyes can tell you. They are the windows of the soul.

By simply understanding what to look for by reading the book or taking a course in Iridology you can look into a mirror and using the map in the next illustration see the main blockages.

Kirlian Photography

The next photo is a leaf that was put in acid and pieces of the leaf had holes in it, leaving the skeleton. Still the leaf showed an aura or energy of the leaf, showing the leaf to be still alive for some time afterwards even though it had been taken from its host tree and bathed in acid.

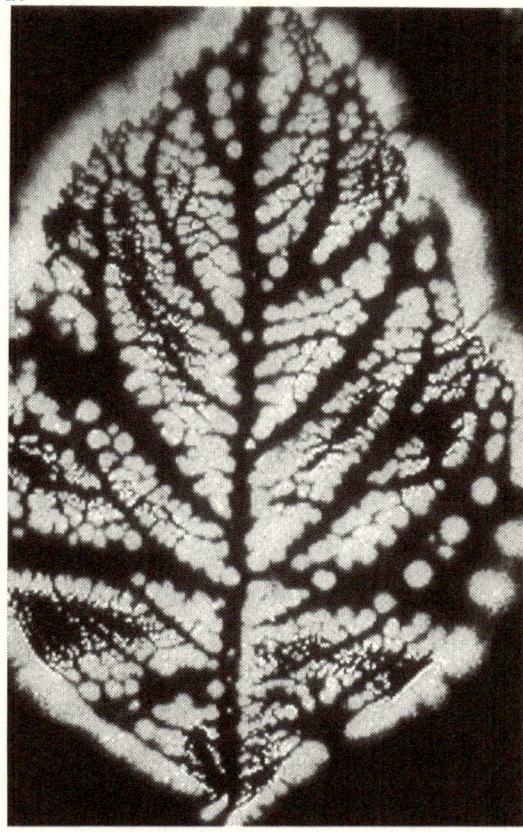

This leaf photo was taken by Graydon Rixon from Bioscan Research Laboratory and was published in the Wellness Magazine in Sydney. The hand is mine taken at a Health and Harmony show in Brisbane Australia.

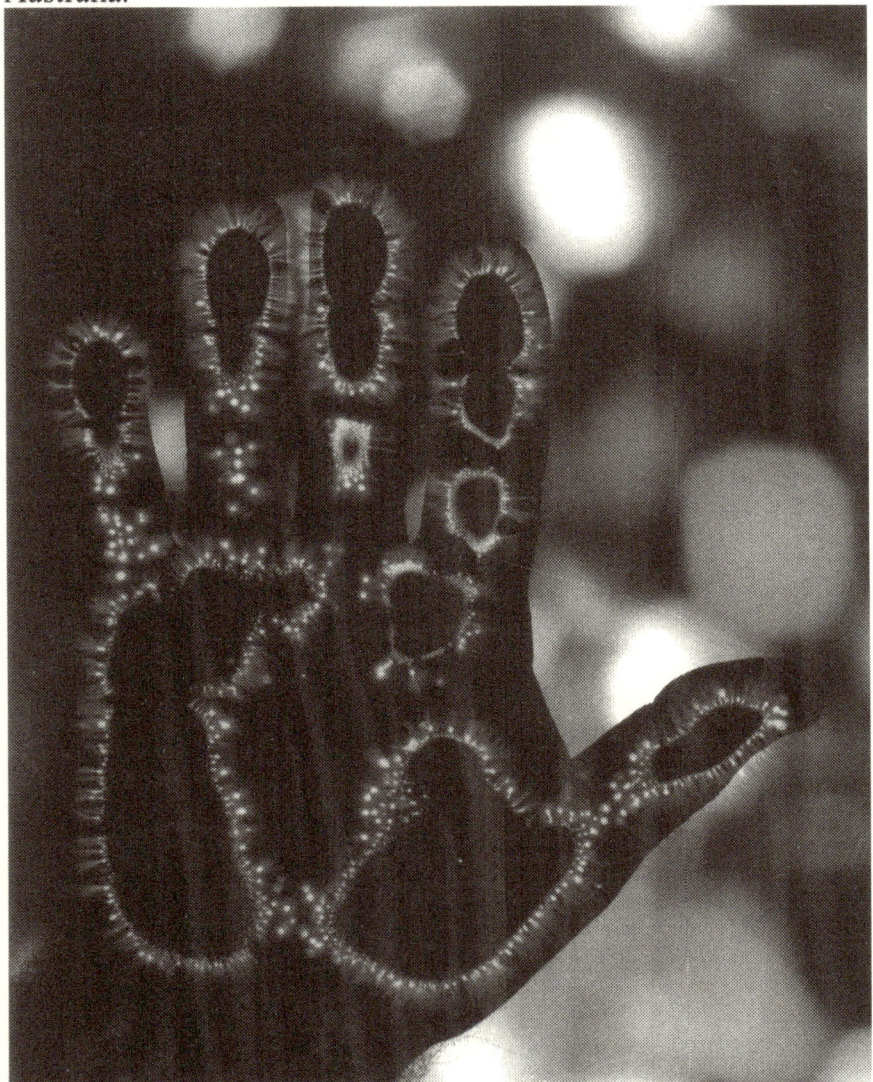

Each and every cell in your body has a memory or a blueprint of the rest of your body, even after being separated from your body.

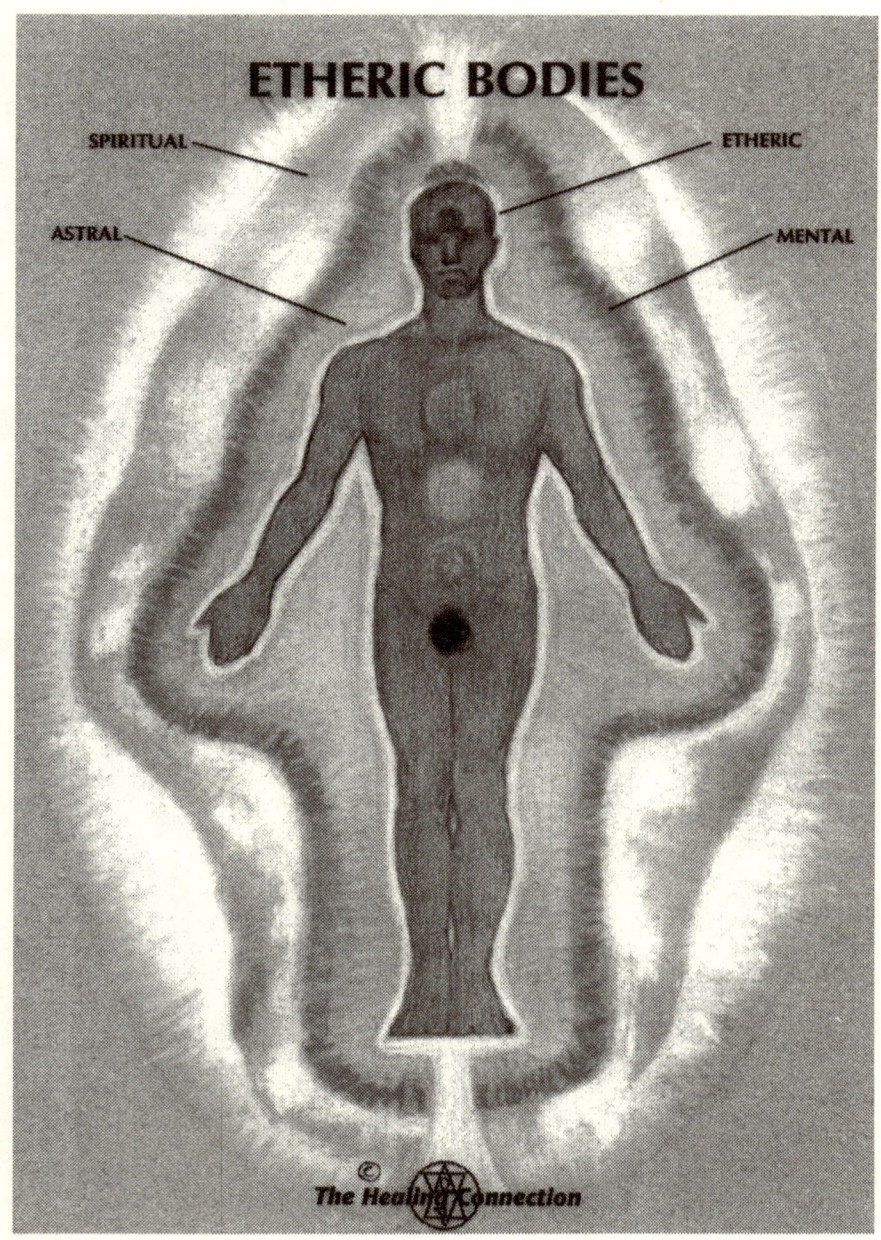

The etheric energy being closest to the body is like the energy field that most people have seen when they are tired at night and have let their eyes go out of focus while talking to someone close by. If you have not seen the etheric energy before then letting your eyes go out of focus while using your peripheral vision the energy is readily seen.

Look above the subject's head in front of a white background, approximately six to nine inches away from their head visually scan slightly to the left or right of the subject. With practice you will sense/see a small energy field approximately a quarter to one inch around the person's head. In the morning or when the person is well rested, this energy will be further out from the body than when he is tired. By letting your eyes go out of focus and concentrating your vision on your own hand you may see the energy up to a quarter of an inch all around your hand. The best place to see this is actually between your fingers when slightly apart.

When I was training to be a healer a group of us in a classroom situation used to breathe inhaling and exhaling all together for approximately 30 minutes while holding hands. We would then break the circle and with the lights out, putting our fingers close together we could see the sparks of etheric energy flowing backward and forward between the fingers. Later we learnt how to harness this energy and send it to some very lucky sick people who when hit by this loving healing energy, didn't stay in hospital long. An observer in a Hospital room once said that the fluorescent light went on above the patient's head at the same time as the group had projected to him. We knew the energy had worked. The light was not plugged in at the time so this caused considerable confusion, much to the chagrin of the nurse who was left in the dark so to speak, as the observer didn't explain.

Here are some of the aura photos that I have had taken at different times to show you what I was talking about. The next Kirlian photos were taken of me at various times in the USA at Whole Life Expos where I was speaking on Health and Healing.

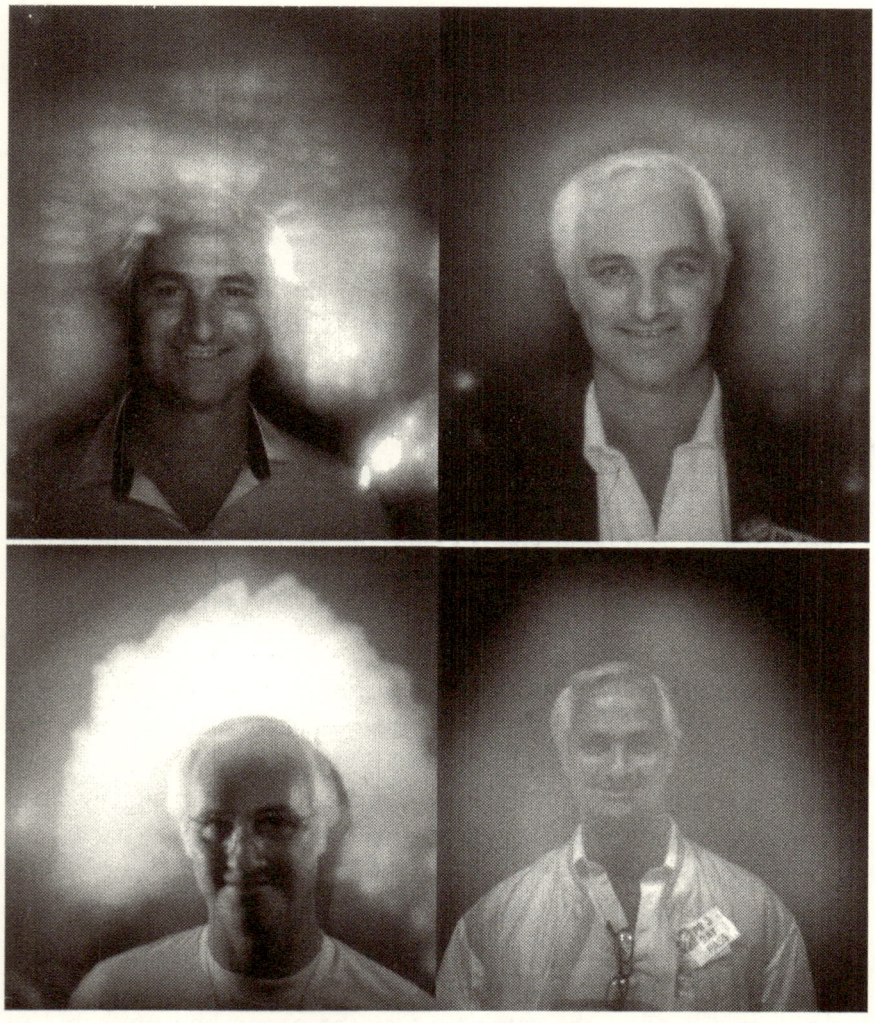

As you can see they are quite varied depending on the stress level and depending on what I had been doing earlier.

The top left photo was taken when I first arrived to talk at the Whole Life Expo in Los Angeles and notice how gray my shoulders looked as I had been carrying heavy suitcases just before arriving. Notice the flare on my left shoulder as I had hurt it prior to arriving also.
The top right photo was taken in New York at the Whole Life Expo as I arrived in the morning on the red-eye express. After completing a two hour healing on a lady who requested my help, I went and had

another photo taken (bottom right) and found much to my surprise I was still surrounded in gold from the healing energies that had channelled through in God's name.

Psychic /Spiritual healing

In the Philippines the best of the Spiritual /Psychic healers state that when operating they put their hands in the bodies of those afflicted with disease. They are able draw the diseased material out of the body as it is attracted into their hands. They believe that God's energy is perfect so by focusing and projecting this energy into one's body all disease must leave.

According to Philippine Spiritual healers David and Helen Elizalde, the body just parts like a sponge when the hands/energy penetrates the skin, and when they take their hands out, the body melds and mends as though nothing happened, leaving a small red mark which fades away really quickly, similar to the parting of the seas of Egypt in Moses' time.
Energy is being open to you from God's loving healing energy for those willing to make change.
The following photo is one I took while working in the Philippines. Notice how the body is open close to the fingers.

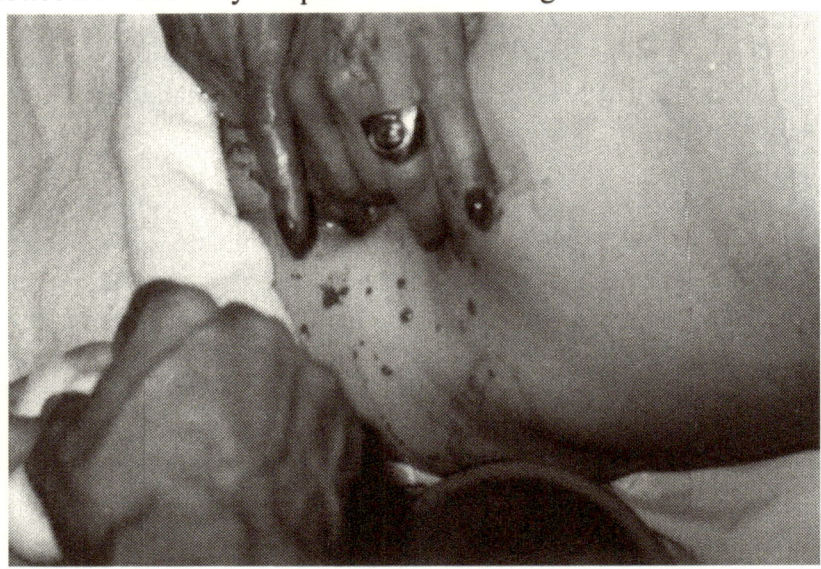

61

Before I hear from you that you have seen documentaries on TV that debunks this theory, I would like to state that I, being of sound and sane mind, experienced the Philippino Spiritual surgery. I know it works from first hand experience and owe a great debt of gratitude to my many healers. I know that I wouldn't be here today had it not been for them and their devotedness to the work of God.

My six weeks in the Philippines was an experience that I will never forget as I witnessed many miracles, and I believe this work and the people who have the gift have the blessing of God and the universe.

I have also read a book compiled and written by 30 professional doctors, psychologists. psychiatrists, scientists, physicists, chiropractors, etc., whose mission was to squash for all time the rumours about Philippine psychic surgery. Unfortunately most copies of this book have been destroyed and the owner would not let his copy out of his sight. It has graphic photographs of many specialist healers working with and on bodies in various places and states of being open with all sort of blood and tissue being pulled out of bodies. Human tissue material that they tested in the Philippines themselves was proven to be human blood and tissue and the blood and tissue material sent overseas to the USA and England was tested and came back as animal blood or suchlike. This happened especially when the doctors stated where the tissue came from.
Sad that such a gift is kept from the majority of people in the order to sell more drugs.

Drug companies earn in excess of $234 million every three days so if greed is their motivation why wouldn't they keep you dependent. We cannot do without drugs or medical surgery and many times I have sent people to a medical doctor for specialist treatment. I believe that it will not be possible to eradicate all drugs, however, where possible and feasible a natural remedy or supplement should be used. Side effects of medical drugs can be nasty!

Most of these intrepid doctors and scientists had operations and the summation was along the lines of:

We do not know how the Philippine Psychic Surgeons do this work but we know that it works and many of us have had work done on our bodies with rather surprising results and quite often full remission. We cannot say it is charlatan as using the bottom line, it does work. Although there does not seem to be any scientific result as to how or why it happens. We can only assume and put this phenomena down to the highly religious state of mind that these gifted practitioners seem to have when working, as they believe that they are a channel for Gods/Universal energies and as such, work as a clear channel as his instrument.

This state of belief attracts some sort of higher power that opens the body and attracts to their fingers the diseased tissue which is then removed by the practitioner leaving a red mark, no scar, and even the red mark dissipates in a very short time.
If any of my family or I need a major operation I would find a good Philippine surgeon to do the work on us first.

Warning: As the Philippines is a very poor country, there are some who do not have the gift but will try and get paid to do an "operation." These people don't have the gift, but it will feed their families for another year with what they get for an operation, if they get away with it.
Please ask around and don't just trust anyone to do the right thing as these people are desperate, as you would be if you were starving.
This could be your life we are talking about so be discerning.

Medical Operations

For those of you who are on the spiritual path it is important to know that sometimes we get so busy and do not slow up enough for our angels or guidance to get a word to us edgeways. Some small operation may be scheduled to stop us or slow us down. For instance if our karma is finished and we are to take a different path then there would need to be some changes done to our energetic system. Please take time to stop, smell the roses, meditate, pray, whatever you do so they can communicate and it also will do wonders for your stress levels. An old friend once said that so many people were in so much of a hurry to get to the top of the mountain that they forgot to stop and enjoy the view.

Having been lucky enough to watch several operations I noticed that before an operation there is a gathering of the clan of angels, guides and the relevant master in charge of the operations.

When your soul comes out of your body during anaesthetic you are taken willingly to gain some wisdom on what happens next, given an update on planetary data while fine tuning changes are made to the energetic /cosmic energy centers /chakras, etc. Your favourite doctor cuts out or fine-tunes the diseased bits of the physical body to his/ her best ability. It can be a blessing if you go into an operation with a positive outlook looking for your guidance and to reunite at those levels.

How often after an operation do you hear of people saying how a person changed so much, for better or worse?

The only drawback can be when if after an operation you feel a lot worse in the self-image department or you seem to gain a lot of weight for no discernible reason.

Using Regressional hypnosis, several clients have complained of exceedingly bad self-images or had gaining a lot of weight after different operations. Most times it has been found that the God in the white coat, (remember his life is in his doctors hands in the subconscious mind) has been talking really negatively about the person as he was having a bad day.

One lady in particular was overweight, self-image lousy and feeling tired all the time.

On regression she found she apparently resembled an ex-wife of the doctor and he had called her a rotten Bitch and a fat lazy useless s--t, plus many other horrible words. The operating doctor stated she was only wasting his time, as she was a low-income operation. After the realization obtained during the regression she shed her weight then regained her confidence and energy levels very quickly.

We must remember that when being open to the elements so to speak, our subconscious mind is like a flight recorder and will use all our senses to look for the fight or flight syndrome for us to use when we wake up or recover. Our subconscious mind remembers everything, and I mean everything, even though we do not remember consciously. This has been proven many times by clients under hypnosis so it is important for your doctor and staff to be positive.

You should have seen my doctor pale when I told him what he said to his head nurse when he thought he had lost me on the table during an appendectomy operation that burst in my abdomen. He thought it was not possible too but is now much more careful to be positive and watch his language during an operation.

Subconscious recording /survival skills could come from the time of trying to survive fighting predators so if we do become conscious before our Sabre Tooth Tiger wakes up, we go into fight or flight and escape. We sometimes think of our bosses and spouses like this too don't we, but this is explained under stress later in the manual.

Subconscious Power /Protection

I once had a client who could not open his hands and they had virtually to be pried apart with massage. He was a rodeo star and in the course of his riding years he went to hospital at least 150 times with broken bones in his body so his subconscious mind closed his hands to protect him from riding a horse and getting hurt again. Ever tried to direct a horse without reins in your hands? After my finishing his massage his hands were supple and the moment he mentioned he might be able to ride in the next rodeo the following weekend his hands promptly closed on him as tight as ever. It was only when he promised to give up riding in the rodeo circuit that his hands unclenched so he could ride normally. His subconscious mind was only trying to protect him, but look at the absolute power of this subconscious protection.

Another time when I was working at a retirement home an elderly lady there was booked in, because she could not walk on one foot. On my day off I massaged her foot and tuned in and sensed her being really tiny and that her body thought she still had glass in her foot. I asked permission to work with her, energised the area and got her to visualise the glass being pulled out by my hand and then healing her wound under the tiny scar. After she stood up and found she could walk normally she booked herself out of the Lodge within a few days. Two months later she phoned me to say as she could not recall ever having glass in her foot so she traced her affliction down in her mothers diaries. According to her mother's writings at approximately two years old she had stood on a bottle and her foot had to be operated on. In her elderly age she jammed her foot in a car door, which galvanised her subconscious mind to protect her from doing further damage to her foot obviously thinking the glass was back and mistakenly tightened all the muscles /ligaments across the scar which caused incredible pain for her to walk on.

Operation Forgiveness

Phantom pains after an operation can be very real and I have found that after operations some people do not heal well, the scars remain hard, and in some these are in the form of electrical happenings, unusual feelings or worse with massive pain in areas that cannot be medically explained

If you have a fist hit you in the same place more than three times the subconscious mind will try to protect you by tightening up the whole area so you will not feel the hurt so much again if the blow is repeated.

Remember that as the subconscious mind is blind and relies on the stimulus it receives as that fist hits, it clenches the muscles round the fist to stop it damaging the organs and retains the feelings/emotions to the memory banks for the next fight or flight scenario. If you are normally in pain before you have an operation and when you wake up and have had something removed you are still in pain from the bits having been cut out. The subconscious mind is in delta as it has been bombed out during the operation with anaesthetic and sometimes does not check to see if there are any missing parts when it wakes up and comes back to reality. When you wake up consciously the subconscious may be confused and go back to the time you had the fist there and clench the muscles across the scar and cause pain. If you have had an ovary and womb out medically for example the subconscious may still send the normal hormones to the ovary areas and the normal electrical stimulus to keep the reproductory area as healthy as it can. So even though a woman may have had her ovaries and womb out in an operation she may still feel at certain times of the cycle that she is getting her monthly cycle. Having no where to go the hormones usually settle into the hips and thighs as this is the closest fatty deposits to defuse it in. I met a guy in Perth Western Australia once who was still scratching the stump of his leg as the gout in his toes still hurt and the gangrenous leg, although surgically taken off, still had the entire energy of the whole leg there. The following cycle is really helpful in these type situations and I believe that as soon as appropriate all patients from major operations are taken through it for the subconscious mind to let go of old patterns. When I have done this before people usually experience a movement right through the operated area like a fine energy checking out what is affected and the phantom /imagined pains stop immediately or soon after and healing is very quick from then on.

Operation Forgiveness
Cycle for phantom /imagined pains.

Visualise or get the person to imagine /remember his body before he had anything wrong with his body preferably at a younger age doing all the things he was able to do with happiness and joy, maybe playing a physical game with someone he loves. Place your hand if appropriate on or over the bandaged scar very lightly and send loving healing energy down through into the whole area visualising peace, love and harmony. Bring his mind forward to the time when he first experienced the pain and then get him to visualise himself going in to see his doctor /specialist to re-experience his emotion of the doctor telling him he is to have an operation.

Now visualising him being wheeled into the operating room and feeling the emotions and thoughts that he had at the time like, will I be OK? Will I be any good again? Will I survive?

Get him to see the doctor cut him open but at the same time get him to visualise God's/Universal golden hands coming down by the operating table, asking his doctor to put whatever is cut out of his body into the golden hands, whether it is bone, tissue, marrow or organs. Do not be surprised if a few suppressed emotions now come to the surface. Allow the tears and be patient as they are healing.

Watching the doctor as he goes about and completes his work and sense a beautiful white light come down from your source and focus in and over the wound putting all the nerves and muscles and ligaments back in their rightful place. Watch your doctor finish and sew you up and thank him for what he did for you as he did the best he knew at that time. Now by looking at all the blood, tissue, bone, organs, etc in the golden hands, thank them and say I am sorry we cannot go until the end of my time here in peace love and harmony but thank you for serving me as well as you did. Bless them for serving you as well as they did and tell them that you will pass them back into the Creators hands for safekeeping.

Ask God /universal energy to take all the bits and pieces back to where they belong in perfect order so that when you pass over you will meet again in perfect order and see the hands going up and back to your source.

After this cycle one will feel the subconscious mind doing a rescan of the affected area with astonishing results for some people.

Past /Prior Life Therapy can be really beneficial if the phantom pains still exist after you have exhausted most of the avenues. Even if the person believes that past/prior life is a load of poppycock or maybe the imagination of the mind, what does it matter as long as the bottom line is you feel better? I have seen clients who after their body has had trauma in the same place more than three times, will either immediately or later regress into a time before where a similar incident took place. Or the person in the subconscious mind will imagine a time and place to get away from a predator in order to escape emotionally. This is usually called a form of soul fragmentation and the job of the therapist is to help the client pull all the parts together by releasing the emotion.

If you can imagine or believe now that you are a whirling mass of electrons, neutrons, etc., all flowing around together held together by your soul, then you need to know that your conditioned thinking is what you have become. See illustrations in the book Hands of Light by the ex-NASA Scientist and Clairvoyant Barbara Ann Brennan.

To be positive is very important and at times know that it's OK to fake it until you make it.

It takes more energy to frown than smile so at least you save energy by smiling.

What your subconscious mind believes, is achieved! This is a reality.

CONSCIOUS/SUBCONSCIOUS MIND

We have a conscious mind and a subconscious mind. The conscious mind is responsible for our reasoning and our intellect, our learning skills, acts as a filter for the subconscious, and will accept affirmations for positivity. Our subconscious mind is responsible for all the automated things that go on in our bodies, like blood temperature, blood pressure, heartbeat, breathing, etc. It is very powerful and can be for us or against us, thinking it is helping us, depending on the negative or positive programming it has received, including from the womb.

The subconscious thinks in pictures, feelings, emotions and symbols, is blind and relies on the stimulus it receives. It has perfect memory and can take either negative or positive programming as the gospels for life. The subconscious mind can be mistaken in the way it wishes to shield you from certain situations. The programming is usually set because a situation was unpleasant or painful, physically or emotionally, when we were too young to know the full scenario and assess the situation accurately.

The saying, You Can't Afford The Luxury Of A Negative Thought, is really relevant to the conscious/subconscious minds.

PRE - BIRTH

All people when regressed back into the womb have been able to tell me exactly what their mothers and fathers have been thinking at the time of their arrival into the mother's body. Whether they were happy, sad, angry or annoyed? even if it was only for a short time, whether they were wanted or not, whether mother was sick, squeamish, hormonal, fearful or not.

Also whether dad was happy, proud, ecstatic, sad, and angry or not. This all has a bearing and an effect on us and our self-image and the quality of our lives. This information gathering for programming continues through all the pregnancy for our subconscious survival patterns. Then during our growing up, in adolescent years each negative or positive is compounded by every rejection we have similar to when it was experienced in the womb.

There is no negative or positive in the subconscious mind. There is only what the subconscious perceives as best for us from its prior programming for our survival.

The subconscious mind takes from your mother what is needed for survival, like blood pressure, temperature, rhythm for your heartbeat, breathing, etc. If you were born in Alaska, to survive its harsh temperature it is important to have a body temperature higher than if you were born in Hawaii so these survival patterns are very important. The subconscious mind dutifully records all it can from your mother's body, mind and brain for your survival.

Let's say mother was really unhappy in her relationship with father. Maybe being fearful about her first pregnancy, hormonally sick, all her hormones changed, she is emotionally unhappy, rather snappy and irritable and not nice to be around. Let's say dad goes away and spends a lot of time at work or with the boys until things get better or is working away.

Chances are, this child will grow up having feelings that to be too healthy is not like mother was, and the subconscious mind will bring about situations to put its charge back to the original pattern that mother and father portray, whether he likes it or not consciously. Even more so if the baby is a girl and is following the feminine pattern.

Another pattern from this mother can be that men cannot be trusted, and can be expected to be angry and sullen all the time, or men will never be there for me especially if father abandoned the child and mother whether emotionally or physically. Inevitably the child will grow up and any time in a relationship, when in love with a beautiful partner will be ever suspicious and just know that the partner is going to leave. Unexplained fears are normally here too, that cannot be explained consciously. Remember that if you fear something happening to you with enough emotion you will draw the experience to you subconsciously for you to release the fear.

E- Motion _ energy in motion again. Be careful what you think, you could get it.

Some of my subconscious subliminal programming was that mother and father were very poor, were known as battlers and worked very hard on the family farm where they both had to work to survive. Not to work well and smart, as they were not taught this.

My father was very frustrated with life, because he always wanted to be a lawyer and as he had to leave school and help on the farm at an early age he hated the farm with a passion as the depression had destroyed his dream for life. When war broke out he was sent off to the home guard and was away for a few weeks. Before he left, my mother and he had a fight about sex, as my mother was concerned about losing me as she was not meant to have any more babies and at such an advanced stage she chose not to have sex with him. My mother has confirmed all this.

My father apparently lost his temper, became very vocally violent and so the whole time he was away, my mother worked extremely hard on the farm so he would be pleased when he came home, and overworked herself while heavily pregnant. It was not possible to get farm help for her during the war,

My patterning in the subconscious mind was that as growing up I had to be big and strong to defend myself and could not trust men, as they were violent. This was confusing for me as I felt it was my right around females to swear and I quite often did and would then feel embarrassed because this conflicting behavior I had picked up from my dad at such an early pre-birth age didn't feel right.

In relationship, for instance in my marriage, even though I knew my wife would go away shopping or visiting with my blessing consciously, I always had the nagging fear she would take off, have sex with someone else and never come home, or have a bad accident. I always had to over please her in my mind. I don't think there was ever a time that she left to go anywhere without a small argument and she eventually did go off with someone else as it was what I feared most and this became an actuality. Can you see the parallels?

Any time we had too loving a relationship I would think of something little that was annoying to me and bring it to her attention feeling safe in the loving feelings, so we would end up in a emotional fight. The family pattern I had picked up and was running was NOT LOVE but one of disharmony and negative attention.

I always had to be in control of all situations, including the finances, and the confusion for me was getting angry and uptight, squashing anger down under enormous control. A mammoth effort was needed to stop out of control behaviour that I had seen a lot of from my father when younger, as his father had. The more I squashed down my anger, being a good Mr nice guy and controlling my anger/temper at all the injustices the more my wife got angry and out of control.
If only knew then what I know now.

This eventually caused enormous stress in my mind and body, which developed into stomach ulcers, back pain problems and heart problems later, and divorce! Any time I saved a lot of money, my car would get mechanical problems or maybe a small crash, ill health would manifest in me or my family, so I spent my money and was poor again. Remember, my parents were poor / broke and battlers. In my mind I had to always work hard, was always tired and had a hard time relaxing without feeling guilty. Subconscious family patterns, YUK!

During a hypnosis regression back into the womb my therapist helped me choose the positive patterning I wanted to run as a survival pattern. My life has been much less stressful since and I now enjoy much better health.

For your own health and sanity find a certified Hypnotherapist, to take you back into the womb of your mother and get help with reprogramming. Remember, it is written that the sins of the father and mother are passed down to the next generation. This is what I believe is meant by the Biblical phrase. It is really surprising how depression and dis-ease disappears really quickly when the subconscious takes on a new programming of health and harmony as being our birthright.

PARENT BASHING

I do not advocate parent bashing. At the time we were growing up, with what they knew, on what they had been taught, our parents did the best they knew how. I chose my parents for the lessons I came in to learn as you chose your parents for what you wanted to learn. Sometimes I think that maybe it was to gain strength, because we needed strength to survive and help change the destructive world patterning. In meditation one day I was told, Know that you choose your parents for all the lessons you have come to learn, like your children choose you for all the lessons that you have chosen to go through.

Sometimes our expectations of our parents exceed what they are capable of. That does not mean that they need to be denigrated in any way shape or form, for whether we like it or not they did do their best. Remember that if you put your parents on a pedestal they will have to fall off as your expectations will always be too high. Forgive them for not reaching your expectations and get on with life. Accept your parents as they are warts and all, as you did not have their experience growing up. Choose or make another family if you like but get off their backs, or expect your children to have to higher expectations of you and repeat the same things to you at a later time.

When you point the finger at someone, there are four fingers pointing back. DUCK
There but for the Grace of GOD go I.

HYPNOSIS OR HYPNOTHERAPY

This is a subject that used to scare me when I was young. I thought that the hypnotist was bad and could take over a soul and get a person to do all sort of things that were not in that person's highest interests. I can still clearly remember my Mother saying to me while pointing to a flyer on a shop window, never go to a hypnotist as he could take me over and then I would have to do his bidding and never be able to get away from him. The hypnotist at that time obviously was good at stage make-up and the flyer looked positively evil so as an impressionable kid it was really easy to believe what was being said.

This was really compounded when my father heard from neighbours that a nearby town was putting on a hypnotist show and the hypnotist was really good. Dad could not resist taking us all as a family to the stage production but put the fear of God into us beforehand.
We were told not to look into his eyes and to watch what was going on for our own education. To see a family friend go up on stage and make a fool of himself by quacking like a duck under the hypnotist's control was scary for a six to seven-year-old. Even more so when he had sat near me and on returning to his seat from the stage with a prior induction command he also performed next to me. After he sat down, he suddenly leapt to his feet and started to sell popcorn with a fervour that was not at all like this normally quiet and reserved person. I was freaked out!

I know everyone has the right to make a living but I do not agree with the use of such a valuable healing tool being used for public spectacle. In the hands of a hypnotist with so much going on stage at the one time, it is easy to use wrong words by mistake, which can cause incredible self-image problems. This has been verified by disturbed people who came to me for deprogramming after hypnotic stage performances. Hypnosis needs to be very private in a quiet conducive surrounding.

Thank God I worked through my fears of hypnosis by studying, reading many Hypnosis books and researching the mind and how it works. Using hypnosis has really changed my life and many other lives for the better. There is still no other way I could have released all the blocks/barriers to my self-growth that I have done to this date. Every day survival was like a major internal battle and accessing some of the unknown fears I carried provided sheer relief of knowing I was not mad or deranged. Living with what others negatively told me was only in my mind and imagination was pure hell. In actual fact they were right, it was in my mind but the ordinary medical methods did not make my life any easier to live comfortably without massive tranquilizers. The quality of life I was looking for and wanted was obtained because life was unbearable the way it was, and I knew it could not have been any worse than it was. This acquired desperation gave me courage to investigate hypnosis. It was either that or kill myself in a long slow death and I chose to live.

Isn't it amazing that when we don't take notice God puts us in a situation where we have to get over the hump or suffer with all sorts of pain. We don't want to move out of the rut we think we are comfortable in and feel we know, which rapidly becomes a grave.

It is very important however to pick a certified hypnotherapist whom you feel you can trust and are comfortable with. If not, choose to leave and find someone you can be comfortable with. It is important to find someone who does not remind you of an old perpetrator from childhood, if there was one. This can also be scary for the therapist when this happens, and the client is not aware of this prior to the session.

Hypnosis is a very natural process and is highly recommended. In the sleep laboratories it has been found that our brain/mind operates on different frequencies during different stages of our life/sleep periods and this changes depending on what we are doing in dream state at the time. We are all energy again.

Let me explain the different frequencies, as I understand them to be.

Beta

14 to 30 cycles per second depending on how stressed we are is the highest on the scale of frequencies. The higher these frequencies climb the more risk we have of breakdown. In other words if we do not take notice of our stress levels and do not get adequate rest, the frequencies climb too high and then the subconscious mind takes over and gives us a breakdown. This will enforce a rest in the delta level. The subconscious mind will take us to a level of consciousness where we are too weak, we cannot work, as the fail safe mechanism comes into play.

Beta comes into play more and more when we develop our intellect around the time of puberty and as long as we get adequate rest and don't get too stressed we will stay at a reasonable level. Meditation and prayer are some of the ways to monitor and get our brain rhythm levels down to the creative healing ALPHA level.

Alpha

7 to 14 cycles per second. This is first recognized and evident in children from approximate ages 3 to 7 years. It is a really creative time when most children learn a whole new language, and from what we can read in the latest publications, can even learn two or three languages quickly and easily. Try that when we are in the beta level at an older age without the use of self-hypnosis and unless you are a linguist it is nearly impossible for most of us to do it with comfort and ease.

The alpha level is where the body can heal really quickly, and really creative ideas can be accessed in this level. As adults we mainly operate in the beta level during the day, except for when we are on the toilet, in the shower or when driving, which by the way is when most people get their really creative inventive ideas. We have, when we sleep, approximately seven periods of time in the alpha which shorten as the night progresses.

The most remembered time of this alpha level is when retiring for bed and all is quiet, just before falling asleep. If someone calls you or knocks on the door, and you know it is not urgent, it is so comfortable that you really don't wish to answer or get up to answer the door. Another time is when you may be sitting in front of the fire watching the flames and a small spark flies out on to the carpet. You notice it but have a difficult time to get your body moving to get up to put the spark out. It's like breaking your mind out of a trance to get moving again. We can normally use these times to sort out our day's planning for the next day, and many good salespersons have developed the alpha techniques of the mind through meditation or hypnosis to be more creative and efficient, while keeping stress levels down.

First up in the morning when we are awake and we can hear everything that is going on but we are just too comfortable, calm and peaceful to move. Another time in ALPHA is while driving a car. You wonder how you could possibly have turned up at your destination and not noticed a lot of what was going on the highway. Maybe you missed your turn. "Where was I"?

Theta

4 to 7cycles per second. If you are woken up sharply by someone when in theta, you feel out of body, really rubbery and will need to go back to sleep to re-enter your body. You feel as though you are misaligned, and you are dreaming in the dream state. It is a time of slowness where time doesn't matter. In other words, if someone

is talking to you in your dream it seems as though they are taking forever to say something simple and time has no meaning.

If you are running in this dream it seems as if you are just floating along similar to the astronauts on the moon landing. Hypnosis seems to work between the alpha and theta levels depending on the subject's levels of susceptibility of induction. In my opinion the theta level is the place where deep subconscious patterning is found by hypnosis. It is possible to access this level of bliss state using meditation but because of the timelessness it is hard to make changes to yourself. Because of the slowness and the feelings of "It really doesn't matter as I have forgotten what I reached this level for now anyway so since I am so comfortable I will just enjoy and maybe do this project tomorrow."

This is where hypnosis is invaluable as there is always a voice to lead you and stop any avoidance in the mind. The subconscious mind will avoid and shield you mistakenly from emotive pain at times if it can.

Delta

Operates at ¼ to 4 cycles per second and is the lowest of the frequencies. This is where your mind will take you when in comatose or breakdown or in an operation situation. You are now in survival mode as all your circuits have blown and you need to rest and regenerate. Children in the womb spend a lot of the time in this frequency as they form their bodies. Closest to nature?

A good book on hypnosis that I can thoroughly recommend for those who may be frightened to see a Hypnotist, and wish to do self help hypnosis is Hypnosis For Change, a Practical Manual Of Hypnotic Techniques by Josie Hadley and Carol Staudacher. This book gives a great explanation about hypnosis and practical examples for the do it yourself person.

Examples of inductions are included to make your own radio cassette tape to play to yourself for results over a period of time. Subjects like to lose weight, combat pain, quit smoking, fight phobias, reduce stress, ease childbirth, increase motivation, improve athletic performance, etc. are all included as well as a good explanation for the lay person on hypnosis and how it works.

The book Toxic Parents by Dr Susan Forward is a very good book to process your childhood and life if you still choose not to do the hypnosis route. I suggest you take your time however and do the exercises slowly and with feeling, as this book will unearth some deep-seated memories that you may have forgotten. You may need to take a little grieving time unless you are one of the 10 per cent who never had anything happen to them.

It was in the reading of Toxic Parents that helped me unearth some really deeply hidden shame of what a farmhand did to me at the age of four. At that tender age my subconscious mind shut off the memories as I did not understand nor was able to cope as to why it happened. Nobody would believe me, and being so tiny I was not able to communicate what happened.

With the perpetrator saying I was lying and threatening to give me more and worse if I told anyone it was a very scary time. That incident bubbled and boiled like a boil for years causing many unknown fears about my safety. Gay men were dangerous! I grew up so strong and tough with the biggest butt you ever did see to ward off unwanted attention. When older I accepted what had happened to me and what gay peoples' sexual preferences were. My attack did cause revulsion in me for many years as my training from nature and animals on the farm for this behavior was only used as derision and a put down.

On deprogramming I learnt to release all blame or shame for my life being out of control at the tender age of four. I was amazed at the rage inside me that I had stuffed down, and I am really blessed to find he had died about three years before I brought all of this back to consciousness. Otherwise I think there would have been skin and hair flying and it would not have been mine.

I learnt to release my anger at my parents and my brothers and sister for not being there to protect me in this predator universe. On looking into this part of my life I could then understand some of my deepest fears. I now have some really good friends in the gay community and have worked with AIDS patients in many places including Louise Hay's San Francisco AIDS meetings feeling nothing but compassion for the difficult path they have chosen.

MEDITATION

I believe that everyone with any sort of dis-ease in their being needs to learn the practice of meditation and self-hypnosis. These are different and treat different areas but both need to be chosen to help alleviate pain and help find your peace within.

Meditation will help you contact your source whatever that is for you, and help you become a part of nature. As we are all a part of nature we do have biological clocks that need to balance with nature and meditation is one of the quickest ways to balance these and help us find peace.

One can relieve some pain with meditation but it is not as effective in pain management as self-hypnosis.

A lot of people find meditative peace by earnest, deep, devout prayer. I have been told by priests who have been taught meditation that their prayers are even more powerful after being taught how to focus and concentrate using these tools of self power, breath and the self realization of being human.

If you are still frightened to use hypnosis then meditation with breath techniques is the one for you to work with. There are many free courses on meditation so I suggest you ask around to find which particular one is good, and the most fun. Its not meant to be that serious, and one can meet some great new friends.

When I was taught at the Alpha Dynamics course we used scientific instruments to measure brain rhythms. We had fun by attaching the machines to our heads and hands and when we reached the alpha state a large noise would go off frightening the living daylights out of you and bringing you right back up to beta level again. We learnt to really concentrate to keep the noise going and go even deeper into the theta levels so we could meditate even in heavy traffic if necessary.

The purpose of meditation is to help you keep still and calm for approximately 30 minutes to an hour and I have been told that scientifically one half hour in the Alpha levels equals approximately two hours of sleep. This gives you an enormous advantage if you are needing a lot more energy to complete a job or project and stops all mind chatter so creative ideas on projects flow in to your mind very quickly.

Approximately 15 years ago I used meditation to complete a project of managing the sales of several projects on the Sunshine Coast in Queensland Australia. To complete this job I used to meditate for 30 minutes on waking in the morning and during this time would plan in the stillness of my mind the day's activities and write down what needed priority. Then at lunchtime allowing 30 minutes for lunch and 30 minutes for meditation, I got literally two hours of sleep under my belt and would have a bundle of energy to complete the day's work. On getting home, to stop the negative parts of my day's activities interfering with my family life, I would then do 30 minutes to release the tension of the day. If this was done it was assured one did not fall asleep at the table and could continue well into the night with intelligent conversation.

After I left this agency I was informed by several salesmen that the agency had to split my section into three more sections as the next

manager was not able to cope with the work load and had stress /
heart problems trying to keep up with the work load. Meditation
WORKS!

While in meditation your breathing, heart rate and metabolism will
all slow up and be in a state of rest yet your mind becomes highly
creative. Your body was never designed to take all the stress that we
as human beings have put onto ourselves and meditation will help us
to heal our bodies and those around us by being a calm influence.

No one can complain about the way this world is unless he or she is
at least making the effort to contribute to the peace in the world. It
will only start with you. It's similar to throwing a stone into a small
still pond or lake. When that stone splashes into the lake, there is
a splash and the little ripples of water go right across to the other
side, then on hitting the other side come right back to you. When
you are at peace, your stillness will affect others, who will in turn
affect their friends and family and make this world a better place to
be in. This has to start now and with you. Meditation is a great way
to start.

When you improve at this you can even be in this self-meditative
state with your eyes open while working. A less stress yet highly
creative state of mind and people will never know you are in it but
will sense you being very calm and having lots of ideas.
Following this paragraph is a copy of a meditation that I have used
for a long time and continue to use it as it gives good results. If you
wish to, record your own voice by reading the words in to a good
radio recorder with music playing softly in the background. Please
pay attention to the pause commands. Then you can play it back.
Most people relax more listening to their own voice, so by listening
to the tape using your own voice you will trust yourself.

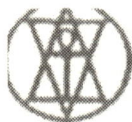 # The Healing Connection
presents
TWO SELF HEALING
MEDITATIONS

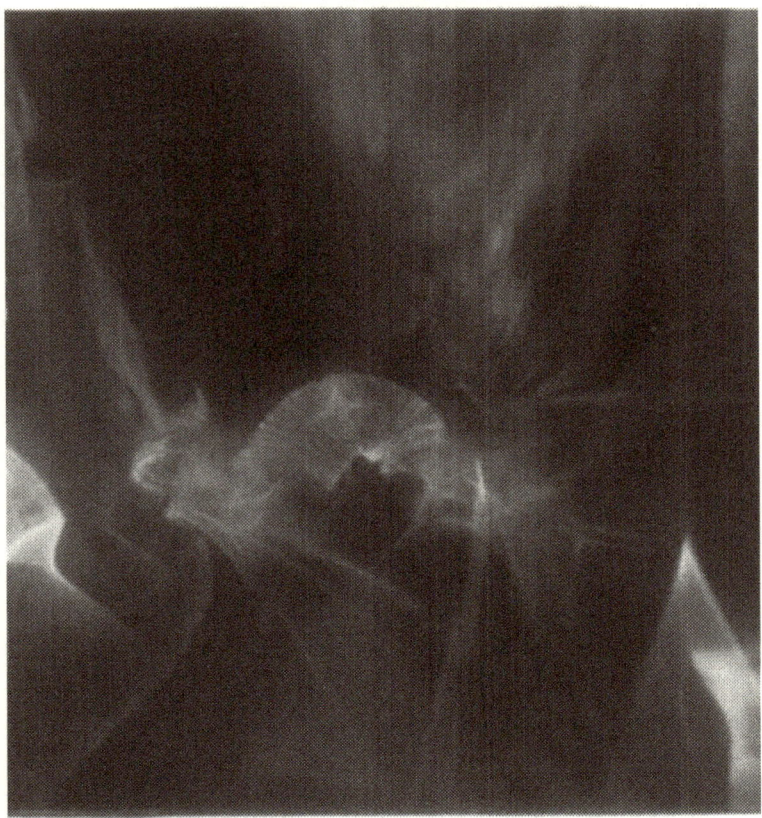

©1990 John Douglas Chamberlin

A professional pre recorded copy of my Self Healing Meditations can be purchased at www.healingconnection.com.au or PO Box 995 Southport BC Queensland 4215 Australia for $20 (includes postage). This CD /radio cassette tape includes two Self-Healing Meditations with Tibetan bells, harps, gongs etc. in the background giving the ultimate in relaxation and a maximum time in the Alpha level that the subconscious mind can use in the one sitting.

SELF HEALING MEDITATION

Find a comfortable position, uncross your arms and legs, close your eyes and direct your mind to the area in your chest known as your heart chakra or heart room.

This room will be set in nature or a favorite place for you, has four walls and no roof and is known in the universe to be the area through which the love, which is rightfully yours from the universe, is filtered into your body. It is also known as a place where you give your love to the universe and other beings in your life.

It should always be peaceful and harmonious and the walls need to high enough to stop anyone coming in here without your permission. The roof needs to be open to allow your guides or guardian angels to be able to come in and give you messages for your highest good from your highest scource.

Walk into your room and notice the color; note whether it is dark or light in color, then ask for a white light to come down from your source, whether it is from God or the Universe into your room. This light has many names such as The Light of Christ Consciousness, Universal Energy, Sumadhi and many others, it doesn't matter what you call it but know that it comes from your source.

Ask and direct this light to act like a huge giant vacuum cleaner and clean up your room from any negativity which may be there and take out into the stratosphere any negative energies, entities, control lines, broadcasts or anything that may not be in your highest interests or good. Take out those who don't have your permission to be there and are pulling on your heartstrings or emotions.

Let this brilliant white light act like a giant vacuum cleaner and suck out all negativity or anything disharmonious to your soul and leave behind peace, perfection and perfect harmony.

I will cease talking now for a short time and you will be able to clean your room so that before we go further the whole atmosphere is a sparkling white or gold or silver.

If you don't see / sense anything now it is important to imagine it, so relax now and enjoy having fun creating as you did when you were a child. The more child like the better.

1/2 minute PAUSE.

Feel now how the whole atmosphere in this room has changed, it is now peaceful and harmonious. Walk now to the center of the room, and there you will find a chair, a cushion or something to sit on.

Sit down and make yourself comfortable, as you will be here for approximately half an hour.

Ask your guardian angels to come in now and be beside you and shield you from all harm as we investigate the meditation levels of the mind.

Next I want you to imagine opening up the top of your head and ask and allow the white light to come in from your scource. Be aware of the tiny muscles on the top of your head as the light passes through them, relaxing, letting go all tension, and feel this relaxation moving like a wave slowly downward throughout your body placing the muscles of your head in a complete and total state of relaxation.

Let this white light flow and move round your brain, and as it goes through sense and see it take away any tension or anything which may not be in complete harmony with you. The darker the area the more this white light will concise like a laser beam and cut all negativity away, leaving peace and balance.

Next let the light go round your eyes, round the tiny little muscles which help your eyes to function properly, and as the light goes round them or through them, see sense and feel all tension leave.

John Chamberlin

Release all pressure and feel them come into a perfect state of focus in a perfect state of perfection and harmony.

Now send the light through your ears, your outer ears, your middle ear, through the tiny nerve endings which transmit your hearing, sensing and seeing to your brain. Check for any blockages and if you see anything dark or gray, force the white light through and through until it is a sparkling white again and all disharmony absorbed.

Concentrate now on your jaw and your throat. Let the light flow round your jaw and throat relaxing all pressure and releasing all tension in your jaw and throat. Gently push the white light through your throat until it is a sparkling white color. Know that your throat is an important area of your physical body for temperature control and metabolism, so make sure it is sparkling clean.

Next, direct the white light to move down your spine starting from the top of your neck and going to the base of your spine bringing perfection, not only to putting bones in their right position, but also to the billions of nerves and nerve endings which lead off to your vital organs or the round discs between the vertebrae acting like pillows to stop compression when you move around.

See the nerve endings and lines humming like a high-powered electricity line glowing with good health and perfection.

15 seconds PAUSE

That's good, now let the white light go into your chest cavity, into your heart space.
Imagine and see the light flowing gently from one chamber to the other leaving behind love, peace and harmony with the valves and muscles working in harmony and perfection. Know that from now on with every beat of your heart, your mind, body and emotions will become more relaxed, and more in tune with nature than ever before. Each time your heart beats you now allow your mind to go deeper

86

and deeper and more close to nature as you wish to experience this peace and harmony.

See this white light when it touches the blood, your life fluid, how it takes away all negativity and leaves peace and love in its place. Most of all sense the light leaving a smile on the faces of all the cells in your body as the light touches them and brings them back to perfection.

15 seconds PAUSE.

Next breathe in this white light --- PAUSE BREATHING IN--- and as you breathe out your stress the first time it might be like the back end of a bus, black and sooty. Don't worry because the more you breathe in deeply the next time you breathe out it will become lighter and lighter until eventually you breathe in white light and breathe out white light.

I will pause for a short time so you can practice this. Remember to breathe in deeply and think of drawing to yourself the strength and power and light of the universal mind. Let the universal power in this white light circulate through you.

I will now pause for a few moments for you to feel this love and energy.

15 seconds PAUSE.

Now let the light flow through all your other organs like your liver, kidneys and stomach. See the light passing through them leaving behind perfection. A perfect balance of alkaline and acid in your stomach so that your stomach and all the glands which control the breakdown and the assimilation of food into the bloodstream, are now in a state of perfect harmony and function in a beautiful, rhythmic, healthy and natural manner.

Push the light down through your reproductory organs taking all tension out leaving behind peace, love, perfection and harmony. If there are any dark spots there, concentrate the light and force it through the spot until it flies off or is absorbed in the light.

Pause 15 seconds.

Take the light now through your intestinal areas, then your hip joints, your knees, your legs, - relax all tension, release all pressure, - the backs of your knees and your calf muscles at the back of your legs, now your ankles, feet and toes.

Push this light through you until you see this white light about six inches beyond the end of your toes. Be aware of how you feel now with this beautiful beam of God's love running through you. Say to yourself "I am a radiant being filled with light and love".

Pause 15 seconds.

Stand up now in your mind and look in front of you, and see slightly above at approximately twenty-two and a half degrees a 12 foot x 12 foot video screen in your room. Walk up the seven steps to it and each time that you take a step feel your whole being lifted up and up. Walk through the video or screen of the mind, whatever you would like to call it, and as you walk through this video you will find yourself enveloped in a white fluffy cloud, where you feel as light as a feather without a care in the world.

Pause 15 seconds.

When you come through the other side you will find your feet on a little white path which winds its way across a valley. On both sides of this path are flowers of all shape, color and variety.

See the wonderful colors and hues, all different but harmonious and oh, smell that fragrance and aroma which fills the air. Inhale - PAUSE AND BREATHE IN ONE IN BREATH - and become one with the atmosphere around you, hear/sense the sounds of nature, drink in and taste the great beauty that completes this whole scene.

Reach out and pick one of the flowers and smell its beautiful essence. This garden is special, as all the flowers and trees here are telepathic, which means if you talk to them they will talk back to you. Mentally say *I love you* and wait for their answer.

Pause 10 seconds.

Did you hear them? PAUSE.

Take the path further now. On the left is a large meadow with tall grass but is easy to walk through and in the distance a small tinkling brook or river on the far side. Walk through this meadow and feel the love of Mother Earth welling up between your feet and toes. Feel the tall grass brushing against your legs and hips and feel this love from Mother Earth pulsing through your body. So much so, you might feel like running, skipping or jumping through this beautiful grassy meadow. Do it if you want. <u>*It's fun!*</u>

Pause. 10 seconds

Now lay down amongst the long grass and feel the closeness of Mother Earth as you look above to the clear blue sky through the tall grass. The grass is waving in the wind as it is gently swayed back and forth by the gentle breezes. Remember the sky is blue and blue is the color of love, so know God hasn't forgotten us and that the whole earth is surrounded by blue.

I will now pause for you to enjoy this beautiful scene of nature.

Pause 30 seconds.

Now get up and walk back onto the path, towards the tall majestic trees in the distance. Feel their strength, majesty and love as you get close to them. Wrap your arms around a big one and put your third *eye or forehead against the trunk of the tree and feel the energy, love and strength this tree gives to you.*

Remember trees have been around for a long time. Feel any negativity draining from you into the ground through the tree.

Pause 15 seconds.

Thank the tree in your own way and then follow the pathway through the trees, tall and stately on both sides. In fact, there are so many and they are so tall that the sunlight only comes through the foliage in little flashes over your body as you walk through.

Keep walking until you come to a beautiful everglade where you see a little pond or lake. See how calm and still it is, peaceful and serene. Look at the water lily flower, that beautiful white lotus in front of you. This is a special place where the lamb and the lion, cat and dog, play together in perfect harmony. There is no friction, only love peace and harmony.

Pause 15 seconds.

As you wish to be as calm and as peaceful as this little scene. Pick up a stone, notice the shape, weight and color then throw it into the lake and watch the tiny ripples go right across the pond, hit the other side, and now return to you lapping at your feet.

So beautiful, so peaceful, so serene.

Pause 5-10 seconds.

Remember this is a special pool and many nice things can happen here so find a nice comfortable seat and enjoy this wondrous scene and see nature at its best. All in balance as you wish to be.
Pause 15 seconds.

How do you feel? Happy, loving, calm. A beautiful soul like you can only be happy here. I will now give you time to breathe in the crisp, clear air, look at the beautiful blue sky and sense the hum of nature with beautiful song birds and butterflies everywhere. Look at the delicate colors of their wings. Watch and enjoy this beautiful, calm, relaxing scene of nature.

Pause 30 seconds.

You can come back here any time you feel the need to be here and have more calmness in your life, but now stand up as it's time to go back. Walk back up the path between the tall trees where the sunlight flits across your face, back past the meadow with the tinkling brook babbling away in the background, back past the beautiful flower bed and then, just before you go through the cloud into your room, pour your love back to all your new friends in this scene. Thank them for being here, then step into the cloud and come back into your room with the four walls and no roof. How does your room feel now?

Pause 15 seconds.

It should be peaceful and loving, happy and serene. Thank your guides or guardian angels for taking you and thank God for this wonderful experience.

You may come from this room and this level of mind whenever you are ready feeling relaxed yet energized, fit and fresh and in tune with life and nature.

End of Meditation

METAMORPHIC TECHNIQUE

Read the book METAMORPHIC TECHNIQUE - Principles and Practice by Gaston Saint-Pierre and Debbie Boater for very subtle subconscious family changes you can make for very low cost and minimum time. This technique combined with hypnosis is a very powerful tool to release subconscious pre birth trauma. It takes very little time to master the technique in my opinion and will release some deep family patterns.

This technique is really great if you have trouble sleeping. Five minutes of rubbing on the side of your foot using talcum powder or oil will slow the energy spinning in the head and calm you down quickly.

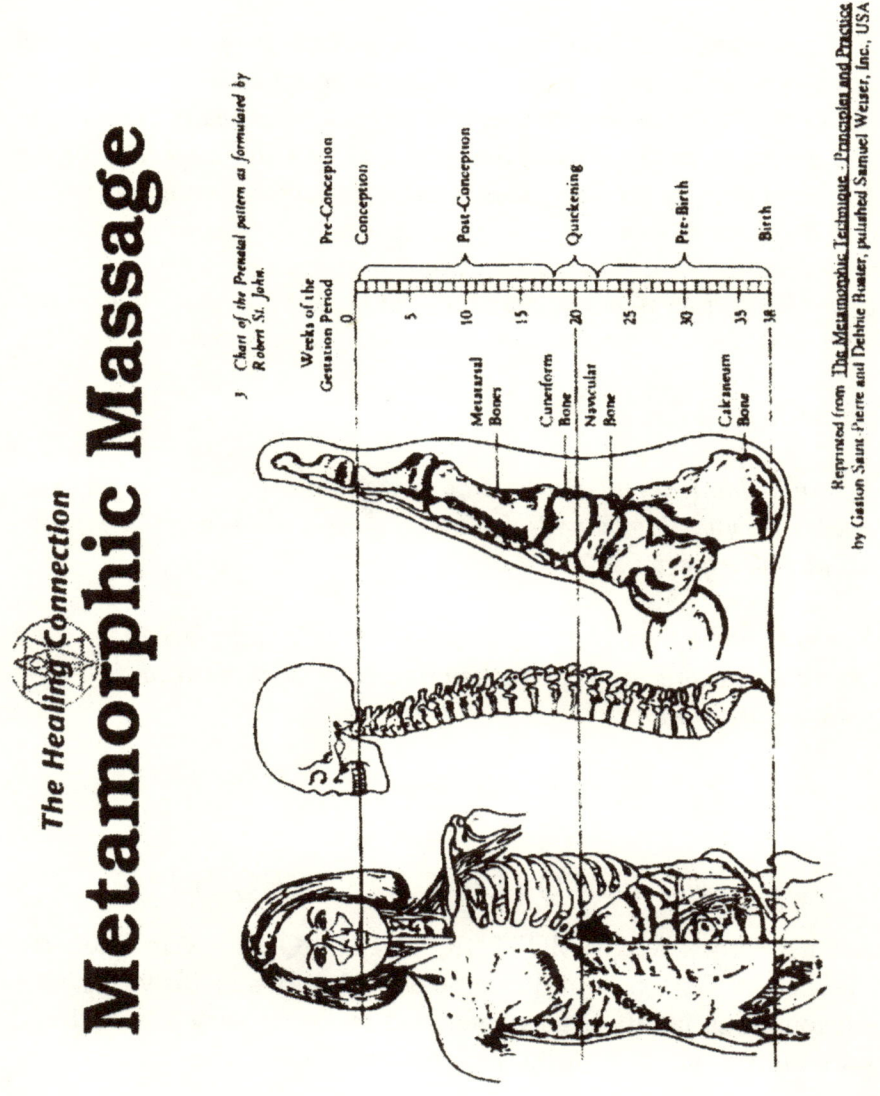

The Healing Connection
Metamorphic Massage

Chart of the Prenatal pattern as formulated by Robert St. John.

Pre-Conception
Conception
Post-Conception
Quickening
Pre-Birth
Birth

Weeks of the Gestation Period

0   5   10   15   20   25   30   35   38

Metatarsal Bones
Cuneiform Bone
Navicular Bone
Calcaneum Bone

Reprinted from *The Metamorphic Technique - Principles and Practice* by Gaston Saint-Pierre and Debbie Roaster, published Samuel Weiser, Inc., USA

Prenatal Pattern

The spinal reflex points reflect also the gestation period from conception to birth. The first joint of the big toe on the outside edge reflects the moment of conception. If we follow a medial line along the bony ridge on the inner side of the foot we find the points reflecting the whole of the gestation period ending at the heel where the Achilles tendon meets the heel bone, that point reflects the moment of birth. The area from the first joint of the big toe to the top of the toe reflects the Preconception State. Conception being at the first joint of the big toe, we have from the joint to a mid-point at the arch the period of post conception, ie the first 18-22 weeks. At the mid point between the internal cuneiform and the navicular bones we have "quickening" between the 18th and 22nd week. From that mid point to the top of the heel bone at the back of the foot we have the period of pre-birth (from the 18th/22nd week to the moment of birth).

Pre-Conception: the movement of the consciousness of the new life towards the moment of conception; the purity of the Life factor is modified by influences, material and non-material, precipitating at conception. The material influences are contributory factors of inheritance parental, racial and human. The non-material influences are the cosmic factors and the human factors created by the human. **Conception:** a focal point in time. Every single factor that decides the nature of the new person is present at this moment.

Post-Conception: formative period. The influences connected with the state of being of the future individual are established.

Quickening: turning point, from self-centerdness to outward exploration and expansion.

Pre-birth: period of preparedness. The influences that will prevail in the activities of the social human being are established.

Birth: period of action or inaction. The influences prevalent then will determine a sense of freedom and fulfilment, or lack of it, in life.

The Metamorphic Association can be contacted at 67 Ritherdon Road Tooting London SW17 8qe PH. 01-672 5951 www.metamorphicassociation.com.uk and they will inform you of the closest office or practitioner to you if you wish to experience this mode of healing

WORD POLLUTION (NEGATIVE THOUGHTS AND REVULSION WORDS)

Every time you have a negative thought, swear or use vulgar words, you set up revulsion in the subconscious mind and weaken your body by up to 25per cent. If you have approximately three to five negative thoughts running round your mind and body then you will most probably be picking up all the coughs and colds, misfortune going around as a form of self punishment, as your subconscious mind will believe that you deserve it.
The most common forms of self-image or psychosomatic illnesses are, overtiredness, depression, lack of energy and being bored.

We implemented in my various Real Estate offices that if any salesman swore or used vulgar language we charged them 20 cents a time. The salesmen and staff became more aware when they swore and how much they did it. At the end of the year we all went out and had dinner out on those who had contributed to the fund. We celebrated on the negative energy changing it to a new positive one.

On recognition of your use of negative words or thoughts it is best to state to yourself out loud if appropriate the words **cancel, cancel, cancel.** After cancelling all negative thoughts each time you have them, enter in your mind and emotions as quickly as possible, **at least three positive solutions** with emotion (e-motion = energy in motion) and **believe** that God or the universe will find a solution for you. Even though you may not see a solution at the time or think the solution is coming fast enough. The overall plan is sometimes not for us to see until we have got the **whole** story from the Boss/GOD/ Universal Intelligence, etc.

Words we use and the power of them affect us. Said often enough these words become a pattern in the subconscious mind and we become the energy of the word in our energetic bodies.

Each word has a geometrical pattern that has an effect on us. One of the greatest of these is the word "OM" which attunes our vibration to the peaceful vibrations of the universe, creating beautiful feelings of well-being in the human mind, body, spirit or soul. It has been scientifically proven now that a chemical change takes place on the cellular level whenever words are spoken.

An example of words producing a chemical change within us occurs when someone describes sucking a sour lemon. This turns on our salivary glands, and either creates revulsion or delight depending on whether or not you like lemons.

Self-talk can be very enlightening if you watch what you say over and over in the next few weeks. It can be fun if you charge the family members a fee every time one of them says a negative word phrase, swear word or you catch them with a negative thought. Then you can go out for dinner on the proceeds and turn the energy into a positive.

Some effects/suggestions
about common words and phrases

Take care	Why? If you wish to live, you have to take risks to embrace life. Life is a school and the only time that you won't be learning to cope on this planet is when you are dead.
Curse it	**Bless it.** Let God be responsible for any injustice. It does go back to those who do the wrong thing by us.

Damn it	**Bless it**. Don't dam anger up in your system
Don't forget	subconscious hears don't and then hears forget.
Remember	will activate the memory.
I forget/forgot	creates a blank wall and gives your mind the command not to remember. By saying **I don't recall at this point**, or **it will come to me later** or **thank you memory for serving me** even when you can't recall something, it takes the pressure off and encourages the subconscious memory to pass the information through to the conscious so you can remember.
Not bad	what is it? Good or bad!! **You either like it or you don't.**
I can't stomach that	will cause gastric problems and maybe ulcers.
I am working my guts out	means a good potbelly coming up here. Change that to **work has been unbelievable!**
My heart bleeds for you	could cause weak walls in the heart.
You make me sick	will make you sick sooner or later.
I am itching to do this/that	rashes, skin irritations coming up.
That burns me up	rashes, hives, skin disorder or hot blood on its way.
That really tears me apart	hernia coming up
I don't want to be fat	make up your mind, what do you want to be?
I want to drop weight	and if you drop something, don't you always pick it up again.
Weight Loss	Use shed or I am shedding excess weight, be positive!
I want to lose weight	when you lose something, don't you always look to find it again.

Pain in the neck	said often enough would give headaches and neck adjustments.
Pain in the ass	will give constipation and even twisted bowel. Actual case.
Pisses me off	incontinence/lack of bladder control/ infections
I am killing time	not in the now. Wiping out the present moment
I am so happy, I could die	what are you living for then.
I can't	you are defeated, **choose** you do it or **choose** not to.
They makes me mad	will make you whatever you want to be, don't blame God if you foam at the mouth.
They make me sick	get a lot of coughs and colds? **Always state that every day in every way I am getting better and better and better.**
They make me sad	they cannot make you anything. This person is not taking responsibility. Sad sorry and usually depressed.

They are dying of cancer etc., they are **living** with dis-ease.

I am sorry	I am contacts the I am followed by sorry equals a negative word or power. Instead say, **excuse me**, as it's not fun to be a sore and sorry human being.
They drive me crazy	losing power here. **Giving your will away. No one can make you anything without your permission.**
I am stupid	lack of self image said often enough, you will forget things, not be able to concentrate and may become stupid.
You are dumb/stupid	said often enough will create a slow person who forgets a lot and is not very creative. If you put a dunce's cap on the person and put him in a

You cheeky little thing	corner that will really give the need for therapy in an older age. Bet on it. don't complain when your child becomes an unbearable cheeky teenager. You asked for it by programming this.
You will never make it	said often enough will provide a really hard barrier for a child or adult to ever be successful.
Could/should	no power here. Don't should on yourself. **Do it or don't!**
I have a problem	**I have a project to work on**, or **my life is challenging at the moment.** Problem is a negative, projects can be solved and challenges like a life crossword puzzle can be fun to solve.

Negative words and phrases destroy your power and if you do not believe me then look up Dr Masaru Emoto on the Internet and look at the photo's of micro cluster water he has gathered for evidence on how human consciousness effects water from different sources and how the power of thoughts can change the molecular structure of water and I believe the world.

Unless you want people you meet to dump all their problems on you, avoid using the words how are you? Use words to empower people and find something that you genuinely believe to be true, to compliment them on. "Your hair is looking great today, do you do it yourself"?

Remember that when talking with other people especially children, it is important to never say repetitively, you're dumb, useless, hopeless, stupid, lazy, ugly, no good, cheeky etc. If these words said often enough, the children/people will become what was said over and over, and will have a drastic effect of destroying their self worth.

The subconscious mind is blind and only relies on the stimulus or information it receives to act upon. Any words said often enough would be acted out in the physical or emotional bodies.

What the subconscious mind believes, whether positive or negative, can and will be achieved!

The subconscious makes a pattern of survival from what you say, be careful what you say.

BE CAREFUL WHAT YOU ARE SAYING.
IT COULD MEAN YOUR, OR SOMEONE ELSE'S
LIFE IS FILLED WITH PAIN, HURT AND SORROW!

Names

Names can be fun. Your name is your call sign and apart from other obvious reasons, if your name is said to you again and again with emotion the subconscious mind will take this as a reality of what you want in life.

I have a friend called Dianne whom everyone called Di, which said again and again as friends and family called her name, sounded like die. She developed cancer. She now insists on being called Dianne and with using other therapies to find out the cause of her disease is now on the road to recovery.

Another client called Bernard, whose friends called him Bernie, was complaining of a burning sensation in his feet and body and is now called BJ.

Douglas shortened to Doug in some overseas countries like Sweden and Denmark and the Philippines sounds like dog. It's not a good feeling to be treated like a dog. I changed my name to John as my full name was John Douglas Chamberlin anyway. My sibling family called me Doug and Douglas. In numerology Doug was like coming up to a wall in life and he would have to knock the wall down using a lot of energy. John however meant coming up to the same wall and instead of bulldozing a way through, the energy of John went round and carried on with minimal effort, a very beneficial change for me.

Buy a book on numerology and if you are not happy with your name change it to what you do like. It is an amazing energy change when you change your name and if you do this be prepared for your whole life perception to change, especially for those close to you who may not have your happiness at heart and may not like the change.

PROGRAM FOR SUCCESS

It's amazing that so many people are so reserved when they win something or find something that the Universe or God has put in their way. The more excited one becomes the more energy the subconscious mind puts into getting it to happen again. Remember to program for success as most of our lives have been used to program negatively unless you were extremely fortunate.

Whenever something happens for you that is good and positive yell out YES! YES! at the same time as you jump up and down excitedly. The arms should be by your sides and hands clenched with the thumbs up and pulled into the sides at the same time as your feet hit the floor or pavement. Do not worry about anyone else. Others will be really happy for you, as happiness is infectious. You have probably just made their day and your infectious glee will give them something to talk about for ages. If you put as much effort into success programming as you do into negative thinking, in a short time your life will be a breeze to get through.

When people answer a question with anything other than yes or no, treat it as no. So if inviting people over for dinner and they give you a maybe, treat it as a **no** and do not prepare anything until a firm answer is given. If it's too late to purchase anything to eat then give them bread and butter, and tell them why. Do not allow friends to manipulate your time by not giving answers. You are better off going to the movies.

When used in a spoken sentence the word "BUT" means disregard all I said before the word but.

REMEMBER. The subconscious mind can understand and relies on truth, and needs a basis to work from.

So the truth is:
Your life has not been filled with happiness or joy in the way of your expectation of how life should be.

Life has not worked the way you really have wanted it to up to now or you would not be reading this manual. When you make changes there are always people who are more comfortable in their ruts and become uncomfortable when you move out of yours and get well.

Remember that the only difference between a rut and a grave is the depth. How deep do you feel you are?

You getting well makes those around you feel uncomfortable as they will lose their grip on you and they will have to question their own beliefs, comfort zones and motives. As you get out from under the emotional thumb, it is unfortunate, and quite usual for some well-meaning relative to try to put you down and get very angry to try to put you back in what he believes is you place in the family, society etc.

Emotionally, some well-meaning relatives may even give wrong advice to keep you more imbalanced than they are, to see someone worse than they are makes them feel better about themselves. It takes courage to make change and it is not easy.

Misery loves company.

True friends support changes for growth and do not put you down. Decide what you want out of life and then with passion and regardless of the cost, **do it.**

Remember this:
One has to embrace living like a lover with passion
And
It's none of your business what other people think of you.

What You Think Of Me Is None Of My Business…by Tony Cole
Whitaker

As far as health and peace of mind is concerned,
You Cannot Afford The Luxury Of A Negative Thought.

AFFIRMATIONS

A positive way of instructing our minds is to say positive statements with energy in motion (emotion) and is by repetition again and again until eventually this new positive information will sink in and be a part of our life. Remember when we had to learn the multiplication tables at school by repetition. The conscious mind filter, on hearing the same thing over and over finally lets the words through to the subconscious mind to keep as a primary pattern so we knew instinctively that 2 x 2 = 4.

In health there are words said again and again that are well meant by our parents or guardians that we have accepted as a program and are not in our highest interests to accept. One example is to say to a child that the sun will burn them, and another is that if our bodies get hit we will bruise. This becomes a belief in the subconscious mind. We have in our blood and bodies exactly the same elements, minerals and vitamins as the earth we live on. If our minds are in tune, our brains can send the required elements, oils or antibiotics to affected dis-eased or burnt places in or on our bodies to fix the problem.

I once knew a lady in Arizona who used to get so burnt with the sun that it became a real problem and she had to dress fully covered down to her ankles and wrists and always wear a hat even inside the house. On regressing her back to the cause of the problem, she saw her mother telling her again and again that she had such a fair skin that she would get burnt, and her mother was continually slathering loads of sun cream on her every time the little girl went outside. Under hypnosis she was told the sun was her friend and was really kissing her skin into a golden tan and was not to be feared. Her body had all the elements to repair any damage done to it prior to this time and would direct her to find and eat foods that may in the future contain minerals/elements/oils that she may be low on to keep her skin supple and moist. What happened next was that when she went out in the sun she needed to re-affirm that "the sun is my friend and is kissing my skin into a golden tan" again and again to herself. Within six months this same lady was laying scantily clad in the sun with her husband enjoying the benefits of being outside with the most beautiful tan she had only dreamed about.

My mother used to say that I always needed to put sun creams on as I had such a fair skin or I would burn. These suggestions worked so well for my friend that I gave myself the same suggestions and within a week or so this began to take effect. There have only been two occasions since that I have been burnt. One was when I happened to be around three or four negative people who happened to observe that I had not put on any sun cream and stated that I would be burnt if I didn't follow their example. I didn't get as badly burnt as they did with all their creams but I did burn. Now I am further down the track in time I understand that my subconscious mind with all its prior programming allowed their beliefs to give me doubts that influenced me on a subconscious level to burn. As long as I am now on my own, or the people I am with do not know that I have not used cream, I have no trouble with my skin burning.

All our muscles are elastic, supple and pliable and it is not natural for the body to dam up or well up blood in an area and stiffen limbs unless it is really damaged. It is really amazing that if you can get to a child who has hurt herself/himself and cover up the afflicted area, while getting the child to concentrate on another area, taking his mind off the afflicted area they will seldom bruise and the pain will be less severe.

Scars from an operation are also a belief and most times when a patients love that part of the body that lets them down in their belief and forgives themselves and others for putting themselves through the pain, the scar tissue becomes pliable and disappears within a very short time. More on this later under operation forgiveness cycle.

Remember now to write down all the words / phrases said to you again and again with emotion that your siblings, friends, parents and guardians stated and you did not question and took to be gospel. These statements were probably passed down to them from their peers and the words controlled them, and have been used to control you as a child, however they may have outgrown their usefulness and don't work in your highest interests. After you have your list of words you will then know what negative energies to release from these words/phrases. They are not true.

A Mantra is writing an affirmation for life that is said again and again and again until it is committed to memory. Just like we had to as children recite again and again the time's tables and our prayers until committed to memory. The following Mantra is taken from one given to me by a professional man who is very successful at what he does. I thank him for allowing me to share.

MANTRA TO RUN MY LIFE BY

- I am always in control of myself and am completely responsible for everything I do. I like myself and I love myself.
- I succeed because I only accept success.
- My desire to succeed is stronger than any problems that will be placed in my way.
- I overcome major problems in my life, and no matter now hard the going gets, I remember that this problem is a here and now problem. Smart working and consistent application will overcome any obstacles placed in my path.

- I am always modest in my self-praise.
- I am humble in my success, avoiding any self-generated public praise.
- I acknowledge the people around me, and always give praise and recognition of their role in my success.
- Alternatively, when things go against me temporarily I accept responsibility for the problems that beset me.
- A problem is a project that with hard work, positivity and time can be overcome.
- I handle ALL matters as they arise **now.** Now is as good as any time to clear a matter that arises.
- I am selective in my approach to life and rely on myself in time of need. I expect no favours.
- I am ethical in my dealings in business and life and assist any that come to me for help to the extent of my ability unconditionally.
- I acknowledge that I am a source of inspiration and hope to many people in the world within which I walk each day. Each day I will generate positivity and inspiration in all I come in touch with.
- I read this plan every day on arising and every night before going to bed, I can recite it word perfect and it is part of every thinking process I carry out.
- I acknowledge that I am a co-creator of the universe and I am capable of carrying out any plan I conceive because the strengths to succeed are contained within me.

Signed:_____

Dated:_____

Two really good books to buy for more information on affirmations on health and the words we say and use are **You Can Heal Your Life** and **You Can Heal Your Body** by Louise Hay. Louise is a really

beautiful lady in every sense of the word who cured her own dis-
ease by using positive affirmations and words. She is to be revered
as she walks her talk and is on the forefront of change helping people
to understand how to help themselves.

MIND GIFTS

Did you know that we all have a different way of thinking, or at
least that's what we say especially when others won't do things as
we want them to. The gift we have chosen to work with depends on
what we have come in to do on this planet, what our mission is, and
what lesson we have come to learn.

We all have these gifts in different orders and strengths, and they are
sometimes in a slightly different order than for other members of the
family so you may be putting yourself down unnecessarily for not
communicating as others in the family wish you to do.

Some mind gifts have a lot of trouble communicating with other
different mind gifts most of the time especially when out of balance.
Let's see how you fare.

TYPES OF PERCEPTION

1. **Visionary Type**: individuals with this type of perception
   generally have a photographic mind. Once they see the picture,
   names, dates, places or events can be recalled with ease. With
   this type, seeing is all-important. Understanding is based on
   seeing a clear picture of the subject or task they are about to
   embark upon. Good organizers when the overall project can be
   seen. They are strongly influenced by pictures, illustrations
   or demonstrations and usually love the movies, TV etc. that
   can be used as an escape. When out of balance or unhappy,
   they tend to sulk or disappear into themselves. They often
   see details missed by others, tend to become perfectionist,
   are neat in their appearance and expect this neatness in
   others. Everything must be in its perfect place to complete
   the picture and they need an attractive working environment.
   Individuals with this sensitivity prefer to transact business in
   person, especially in the initial contact. In communication, they

need lots of words to conjure up the pictures in their mind and brain and are quite often seen waving their arms around drawing the item they are describing. People describing something to them may think they are a little slow. Do not believe this, it is not necessarily so. Once they get it they have it for all time. These people have a photographic memory. Just upset one using this mind gift and you will learn all the bad things you have done to them for as long as you have known them. It's not that they only remember the bad things, they can recall item by item, picture by picture. These people can recount and give you an exact description, a three-hour episode of a two-hour movie they have seen.

Body signs include soft skin, usually long fingers and toes, high arch in the foot, body slightly willowy in shape and usually trim, taught and terrific as the picture of themselves has to look good. These people take a long time to get over a relationship, as at the time of falling in love they draw the picture for life with the house, the car, the kids, etc. When their partner leaves the picture they feel their picture for life has been destroyed. They take it really personally, lose energy and get depressed until they redraw their picture for life again. Very creative people with color who make great decorators in creating a color coordinated home, flowers, cosmetology or dressing and makeup on their own person. Cannot bear to wear the same thing twice so will be really creative with scarves and such to make an outfit look different. Usually can see their guides when taught how to and have colour in their dream state.

2. **Intuitive Type**: individuals with this kind of perception are born leaders. Their intellect is highly developed with a keen sense of discrimination. Knowing and understanding are essential before they can comfortably move into action. However, when they make up their mind to do something, they are interested in the big picture or overall system. Quality is important to these individuals and their work is carefully thought out. When growing up, quite often they will annoy people with the asking questions starting with the word WHY?

People with this sensitivity cannot work effectively under pressure. They tend to become impatient with less organized minds and cannot be regimented. They are self-protective, generally introverted and introspective. They may find it difficult to communicate ideas to individuals of the feeling/ visionary type as they will not have the patience to do so. If they are out of balance, they tend to put someone down in the company of others and usually are quite sarcastic. When unhappy, it's best for them to be creative: cooking, gardening, painting, etc. They need to keep their hands busy to bring the energy out of the head into the hands and slow down the intellect.

Individuals with intuitive perception have an active creative ability. Inactivity or routine work quickly bores them. They are influenced by the thoughts of others and become depressed in a negative environment. This is a very powerful mind when it is positive and balanced with constructive feeling, is generally very good in organizing in business and usually has a great memory for phone numbers. These people are also the early risers, at the crack of dawn, anxious to start the day and will want to know everything that goes on. However they usually go to bed rather early too as this is how their energy flows.

They are usually able to talk with their Guardian Angels/Guides/ Spirit as they hear their voices and usually the answer is so quick to come back they will doubt the voice, thinking it's their own imagination. First thought will always be right for this type and the second thought will be their conscious mind answering with all its conditioning. Body type for intuitive is usually compact and they are usually competitive sports persons. They have long side straight fingernails and toes with no flare in the nail.

3. **Feeling Type**: Feeling individuals are extremely sensitive to the environment and especially other individuals. Patience is one of their virtues. They are usually very devoted to a cause, company, family or another individual. This type mixes easily

and works well with others. With praise they will usually overwork because of the feeling of being needed, wanted and important. They like to work with their hands and enjoy detail work. Feeler types love to touch others as they gather their information from touch. This need to touch can be misconstrued by partners as promiscuous, however this is just how they get their communication. If your partner is a feeler type he will know that you are in a bad mood long before you even get in the door of the house and you will only confuse him by saying you are fine, when that is not true. Feeling types already know the truth, as they are extremely sensitive. Out of balance, they will say don't touch me, but in actual fact the sooner they have touch or a non-sexual massage the better and quicker they will restore balance.

Individuals with this type of sensitivity are excellent followers, but generally are not a leaders as they are frightened to do the wrong thing and take charge until they know the job back to front and inside out. However they need a blueprint for everything they do and need to know where their responsibility begins and ends. Because they automatically translate thoughts into feelings, they cannot take excessive criticism or pressure and are wounded emotionally really easily. It is very difficult for this type to forget or throw off hurt and will defend a member of their family to the last if they think they are in the right. They never forget a person who did them a good turn, and are very loyal. It is beneficial for this type to develop their intuitive abilities. Feelers do not, and will not get on with prophetic types as they do not like con types, dishonesty in any form especially when it affects someone they love and cannot take unkind criticism as they turn what is said into a feeling. However, they respond very well to praise.

Body type: is usually well rounded, strong, with short, stubby hands and feet. They are good with their hands, love kids, are homebodies and protective of the family unit (they live for it). Spiritually feel their guides. First impression gut feeling is always 100 per cent right if they listen to it and go by it.

4. **Prophetic Type**: individuals with this sensitivity who have a healthy, balanced orientation to life often become outstanding executives. Because they have a strong concern for the future, they plan ahead. Although they lack the compulsive drive of the intuitive type, they can carry projected programs through to successful completion. People respect these types of leaders because they are very responsive to ideas and feelings of others. If they find themselves under pressure, they can logically appraise the situation and take steps to correct the problem. These types while growing up tends to be a **smart-asses** – always KNOW it - they don't know how they know, they are good ideas people to work with. They may be moody if they let other people unduly influence them. They can be very critical and manipulative as they have the ability to read minds and may feel the need to control the people under or around them. People of this type tend to spread themselves too thin and take on more work than they can effectively handle. These people have a passion for order and try to keep tabs on all that concerns them. Through order, personal control and personal direction, these individuals maintain a necessary sense of security. Finally, these types must be creative or they become very irritable. They quite often come up with ideas approximately two to five years BEFORE the general public can accept it.

The prophet's only patience is right now - **it's got to be done now, or yesterday!** They love a challenge and make very good sales people. Prophets don't get on with feeler/visionary types as they are too slow for prophets to instruct and very few have the patience to instruct them, but they are good at delegating to get time off for themselves. They can be quite unreasonable with time constraints, if they want something done in a hurry, and can almost be bullies at times when out of balance. These very strong minds can often read another's mind without knowing it, and will if out of balance invade to get the job done or to get their own way. They expect 100 per cent of themselves and get bored quickly with a job when they get to the top. They feel as though they are a failure if they don't win and second place is not winning. When they get down they need a gigantic kick to get back up on top again and this can be hard for their partners to as they can get so negative. Children growing up with this gift of prophet are very precocious, have no patience and when they have done something like a jig saw puzzle will seldom not do it again as they have already done it, conquered it and will annoy others in the family to relieve boredom.

The body type is generally short and fat or well muscled with a thick neck and spade shaped nails. As the name suggests, being prophetic, as they open up to spirituality and take up the spiritual path, they quite often pick up the accidents or negative aspects around the world which confuses them for awhile. Regarding Guardian Angels/Spiritual guides they will just know their guidance is there and what they are saying. It's a knowing, similar to the intuitive mind.

5. **Master**: one who has the self-mastery and balancing of all the gifts or types. We have all the mind gifts, we just have to balance them so we can feel fulfilled, worthy and in tune. Usually we have one gift in the pattern first which dictates the personality for this lifetime. The two stronger mind gifts are prophet and intuitive. The second gift is usually one of the softer gifts like visionary or feeler. The third and fourth is in any order depending on the person and their mission. The only time, to my knowledge, the two mind gifts of prophet/intuitive are together is when the soul has a really special job to do like president or leader of the country. This cuts out a lot of feeling and the person can get the job done without worrying about the consequences or self image feelings as much as others would. **NOTE**: Some children can grow up under the strong influence of a parent who are so strong in their gift that they emulate them especially if they are the winner in a relationship, and so grow up to use the wrong gift and become out of balance. This will create mental confusion until they get back into balance with their first main gift.

Toes and fingers are shaped by energy. As the aura energy leaves the body via the fingers and toes the energy shapes them so the mind gifts are usually represented in the following shapes:

PROPHET   Spade shaped nails, wider at the end of the finger than the quick or bed of the nail. Wider vision.

INTUITIVE   Straight edge nails. More tunnel or straight vision like a concentrated data orientated computer brain.

FEELING   Large fingers and toes with fleshy edge to nails. Very strong physical body.

VISIONARY   Long fingers and toes, usually has high arch in foot. Thin willowy body.

MASTER   Balance of all of these. This is to be used as a guide only as we need to take in the overall picture of a person.

Remember to understand how someone is thinking today and how best to relate to them:

The Prophet - KNOWS - says I know - trances really well - makes a good channel. Likes to get right through and find out the truth about a situation - Loves a challenge. Great salesmen, managers, leaders.

The Visionary - SEES - says I see that - that looks good - make good clairvoyants - Have photographic memories - are very artistic.

The Intuitive - HEARS - is action orientated - makes a good clairaudient- great organiser. Asks lots of questions. Data orientated.

The Feeler - FEELS - says that feels right - that feels good - will be a sensitive - good at Healing/Automatic writing/Psychometry - good artists - normally very good with hands.

These mind gifts are really beneficial to learn if you are in a selling occupation, as you will know how to relate to the person well. There is another skill to learn. Remember God gave us two ears and one mouth. Please take the inference to listen twice as much as you talk if you wish to ascertain another's way of thinking for better communication.

If you wish to find out what your mind gifts are or to have Blockage Discovery Counselling, contact the Americana Leadership College Inc. On 1-800-336-8008 (USA) or write to PO Box 4992 Washington, DC 20008 to find out the address of the closest practitioner to you. They have some good programs to experience, which are very empowering.

CHOOSE/TIME LIMITS FOR SANITY

If you are in a place you don't want to be in, set about to change it or choose to be there for now and set time limits with reviews. The subconscious mind does not allow one to be comfortable in a boxed in situation for long periods of time without enormous amounts of stress.

At one time in my life I was a very successful Real Estate Proprietor/ Broker in Land, Houses, Motels, Hotels, Commercial, Industrial, Special projects, Commercial and Residential Management, Auctioning, Residential and Commercial Rentals, Insurance and Finance, etc.

Also a Certified Train the Trainer for the Real Estate Institute of Australia for Management and Sales training,

I had owned, built up and sold Real Estate Agencies, worked with the largest and best of the Major Real Estate Companies and Agencies in Australia. Now that I had trained as a Train the Trainer for The Real Estate Institute of Australia I wanted with all my being to be one of the best in the Real Estate field and to retire early to help my children be successful if they wanted help.

After going through my divorce, being left with my two boys to bring up, and having to face the knowledge that in this game of Real Estate I was a workaholic, I decided to make the change to a better life style and have more time off with a new partner in my life when this eventually was to happen. This was really refreshing for a while and then I gradually got back to working seven days a week and not giving enough time for my wife and children as the economy worsened and sales slowed. I was stuck in the old patterns of survival again.

I had borrowed too much money and after a change of government in Australia, Real Estate finance became hard to get. My company's Real Estate business gross sales went from $1,000,000 a month to $100,000 a month to $65,000 a month the next month to $25,000 the following month. The down spiral in the economy happened really quickly.

After several years of struggle, transferring money from one account to another to meet my commitments, being very tired one day I asked God to take over my life, as obviously I could not see the whole plan from where I was sitting.

At this time I was working my normal job or maybe I could call it an abnormal stressful job, getting paid from my Real Estate employment, facilitating healing and teaching people anti stress techniques at night for whatever they could afford on a donation basis. Working with the healing energies helped me to release my own stress levels from work as working in the healing energies required long periods in the Alpha levels.

Sometimes I would work most of the night helping people heal to find that most people were just taking advantage of me and did not put anything in the honesty box. I became very disillusioned. Nobody had informed me that for a client to get maximum benefit of healing, it was and is necessary for the person to pay in some form of energy, whether it is money or helping the healer in some way.

Subconsciously the people worked on will not get the full benefit of the healing energy unless there is some form of energy exchange.

Please don't join the hundreds of people who take it upon themselves to run from healer to healer, group to group, giving over your power to others. The buck stops here.

In most cases healers and meditation leaders note and have experienced these types of people, who do not take responsibility and run the excuse that if anything goes wrong with their lives they then have someone else to blame. Most of these people put over good heart breaking stories to get freebies, and then wonder why they don't get well. The universal energy is strict about equality and energy exchange.

At that time I had a local GP who after seeing me himself for a problem and getting great relief, referred people to me for regressions and bodywork. He suddenly stopped referring clients. When I phoned him to ask him why he was not sending clients any more, he said that he had nothing against me or my work, but by referring them to me as they got well and he lost a lot of patients. Even though he was happy that these patients got well, whether he liked it or not he still had his rent to pay. That income dried up for me too.

I meditated every day for approximately 30 - 45 mins in the morning, lunch time and evening to give me the energy to cope. I had been doing this for many years to cope with the stress level and knew it worked. After leaving one job, the manager who took over phoned me and asked how on earth had I coped. He cut the workload into three different sections with three new managers to manage the business because of the stress involved. Thirty minutes in the Alpha level during meditation gives one the relaxation of two hours sleep, so helps in releasing stress.
It's wise to learn meditation to be effective!

I made a decision then to talk to GOD or whoever is or was in charge out there!

GOD, if you want me to be a full-time healer then you are going to have to make it happen for me as I can't see the way to survive as a healer full-time. If you want me to stay in Real Estate then I will do that too, but for now I want you to take over my life and I will endeavour to get out of the way and let **Thy Will Be Done.**

With that thought in my mind I brought what I imagined to be God's golden hands down in my mind's eye and put all my problems into them. My unhappy wife and children went up in the first load. My business and all its associated problems together with my properties that I was having so much trouble selling in the second load so I could pay my debts. Then I put myself in the third and last load into God's hands and said out loud, clearly:

GOD, let thy will be done for me, I will accept with as much graciousness as I can. If there is no change then I am to struggle for the rest of my life, as that will be what you want for me. If there is a massive swing in another direction even though I may not like or want too physically or emotionally do this I will recognize this as your will and I will choose to be there for as long as you want me there. But could I put a limit on this for six years? Boy was I a scared chicken!

What happened next was rather scary. I went to work and lived for each day, hour, minute and moment. During the next week, rather that just expecting as per my perception of what I thought people should do, I allowed the salesmen as much as it was lawful to express themselves, do their thing as much as they wanted to.

I started to enjoy myself, sales went up, and much to my surprise, all my properties sold within the next two weeks. My separated wife decided to go to a smaller apartment, my middle son decided to go and stay with his brother and I got an offer on my business and car which was financed with the business.

I started to get scared as it seemed to be going too quickly for me and a voice came in my head saying, "**Just let go! You asked for help, so now get out of the way.**"

I also had an offer from a really good past life therapist and healer to go into partnership, start a Healing Center, travel and learn more about healing. I had been so bogged down with the how do I pay the bills that it was impossible for me to be in the here and now.

My business sold and I was able to pay all my bills, which I previously thought impossible with a small sum left to split with my separated wife.

I got the message. When every thing looks as though it's impossible then its time to ask God and your Guardian Angels to help.

An Angel during a meditation once said: "How would you like to be literally sitting here on a cloud and not being asked to help? We do want to help and we know we can be of service. That's what we were created for, but humans were given free will, and we may not enter and help unless you ask us. **SO ASK US, PLEASE!**"

Chapter 11 in a Book called The Dynamic Laws of Healing by Catherine Ponder shows a beautiful way to write to angels and change situations if you feel you cannot talk to angels yourself.

CHOOSE EMPLOYMENT

If you are unhappy with your job or your boss, ask for help, use the golden hands, or **change your situation** by leaving or choose to be there for at least another three or six months and give it your best shot.

I have had so many people say during sessions that they can't make change in their life because of the money or what others would say but haven't even looked at the options like sickness and disease. Maybe God wants you to do something else and your time of struggle is past. You have free will so even God will not force you to move if you want to stay in a situation. He will, however, give you an opportunity when your lesson has finished and keep giving you gentle hints until you recognize it and move on.

REMEMBER, that the only difference between the rut and a grave is the depth.

Employers

It's only natural that your employers want a fair day's work for a fair day's pay so give it to them. **Do unto others, as you would wish done unto you.**

If you were paying the bills you would want this too. Time and again when questioning self made business personnel who were complaining of employees using them they acknowledged that they too used the system. Don't steal or abuse the system. If you do you cannot complain if you get used or abused yourself later on. THAT'S A FACT. The energy is very subtle. This was pointed out to me once by a very talented Reiki Master in Sweden when I complained that my Self Healing radio cassettes were not selling as well as I had wanted them to. The Reiki master noticed that I was using copies of radio cassette tapes to play while working. By not paying for his creativity that deserved to be paid for and virtually stealing his prosperity, how could I expect people not to copy my tapes and books and affect my prosperity. I have never copied one since and I now have now paid for copies of music and my tapes C/D's are selling well.

Take responsibility. Don't take the soaps shampoos, toilet paper, towels, cutlery, crockery etc. in a hotel /motel if you don't use them while on the premises. There is no other word for it but **stealing**. The proprietor of the hotel/motel will have to pass on the costs and eventually we always have to pay more for our accommodation as the hotel chain management has to put prices up to cater for this. The manager has to forecast a profit to present to his shareholders who expect a return for moneys outlaid. I have a friend who is a general manager for a large hotel chain with 350 odd rooms under his care. It is unbelievable to see the destructive things people do to a motel room. Treat the room and facilities like your own place and help keep costs down for your kids. Or expect your own place to be trashed later on when you least expect it.

Think before you take something that is not yours as subconscious karma returns quickly. The more aware you become and the faster the planetary energy becomes, the quicker the return. Likewise good positive deeds will return one hundred fold.

Let me tell you a story about this one. A friend introduced me to who I thought was a rather nice lady and we made arrangements to go out the next week. We kept in phone contact during the week so it looked as though we were going to have a great time.
The evening went beautifully, with sparkling conversation from a very witty and charming lady who obviously was very intelligent. After the meal we decided to have coffee which I went and ordered and brought back to the table where we had finished the main meal. On finishing her first coffee she decided to go and get another coffee. When she came back I noticed she had several rather expensive looking chocolate sweets and she asked if I wanted one, to which I accepted and on unwrapping it innocently asked how much they were as they looked so good. She replied that she didn't pay for them. On hearing that I asked, How come, did they give them to you to which she replied , sort of.

By now I was really suspicious and not happy with the explanation, rewrapped the sweet and I dug in to get some answers. The whole story eventually came out that this was a sort of a game to her. I explained about karma and the effects of damage she was doing to herself and her excuse was that she did not have enough money to pay for them as she had just lost her job, and she did this quite frequently. I was devastated as this evening in my mind was down the tubes, so I went over to the cashier and stated that my guest had forgotten to pay for four of the chocolates he had on the counter. On finding out how much the chocolates cost, I paid for them with as little drama as possible as half of them had been eaten although I still did not eat mine.

On the way back to the car to return home she lost one of her best gold earrings as we walked over a bridge. It fell not to be seen again. It was as though it flew off her ear. She was visibly upset but muttered that the clasp was really strong and had never fallen off before. She stated it must be karma coming back quickly.

I might add I lost interest as I felt that I could not trust her, but to her credit, several days later she phoned me and apologized for her behaviour. She said she looked through her life with a fine toothcomb and found that every time she took something there was a drama in her life shortly after it. She learnt a valuable though tough lesson.

If you shirk your work, use the telephone in your boss's time, take the petty cash without permission, or do your personal projects in work time, **it is stealing** and is not your right. All this is recorded as right or wrong by your subconscious mind just like a cassette recorder and it will punish you in some way. If you cheat or steal in any way, no matter how infinitesimal, you cannot complain if you are stolen from or if your health is not in good order as you will have drawn it to you. This energy is so subtle and will be ever vigilant as the earths energies speed up it come back even quicker that before. We have instant coffee so why not instant Karma.

KEEP THE TRUTH AS YOUR GUIDE!

The subconscious mind is blind, and relies on the information it receives, through emotion or repetition, negative and positive programming or influences. It does not have gray areas, only knows black or white. **TRUTH OR LIES! Scary Huh.** When people choose to stay in their employment for another three months or so using choice, the subconscious doesn't feel confined or restricted with no way out. The situation is reassessed and the employment becomes quite tolerable. Other employees in most cases have a turn around in attitudes and have treated the individual much better. Remember the person's subconscious was probably telling other work mates to reflect and give them a hard time, as this was what they deserved.

Know the subconscious mind does not like to be confined in any way and so by choosing to be there wherever you are working, living in life, the pressure subsides and anxiety disappears.
The 60 billion brain cells get focused in the living in the now especially if there is a way out in three to four months or so.

RELATIONSHIPS

If you are in an unhappy relationship, get counselling or talk about it. If your partner won't talk about your projects, or won't go to counselling, then give a time frame for it to happen. If nothing is forthcoming then get out of this dysfunctional relationship and leave until the partner decides to get some help or shows intent on change. The relationship will not get better without getting all the unspoken emotion out and most times, your partner does not believe you are serious until you leave.

I am not one who will tell anyone to leave a relationship, and my sessions are always aimed to pulling people back together by releasing all subconscious programming between them so the relationship is enhanced. There are exceptions to every rule and that is not for anyone or for any therapist to judge, but if any lines must be drawn then the next paragraph is it.

The Indians have a wonderful saying: **Walk a mile in my moccasins before you criticize me.**

If there is violence in the relationship, whether it be emotional or physical abuse, GET HELP! There is no shame and it can happen to anyone so talk to authorities. There are many free welfare institutions around like The Salvation Army, Alcoholics Anonymous, and Women's Shelters that will help and give information on other organizations if their facilities do not match your needs.

Statistics say, it does not get better, so **stop dreaming** or the worst is still to come. Violence, whether emotional or physical will at most times affect you, and your children's health in the worst way. Not only that, if your children are brought up in a violent household in most incidences they also attract a similar relationship as they think it is normal to have violence in a relationship, when it isn't necessary.

If you don't get help from the counselor you are seeing, change your therapist until you find someone who is compatible. Therapists are human too and can be making mistakes by incorrectly assessing the situation because of their own conditioning or situations. Normally I will refer a client to another therapist if I have a problem communicating and most good therapists will if they have the client's interests at heart.

Sometimes it's as simple as maybe I look like someone that was in their life at a younger age who was a perpetrator, or predator. Having blocked it from their memories to cope with life, I know they will not let me know all their hidden secrets if they feel threatened or pursued!

I always used to think a normal family yelled and was controlled by the males of the household. When I was young, women in the family were always the placators and did all the cleaning and cooking. They helped you when you needed help, got pregnant, looked after the first aid and at certain times of the month you tiptoed round them as they got hormonal, angry or uncontrollable. Thank GOD I worked this one out, as it's nice to change the pattern and share the loads and responsibilities. I am proud to see my sons sharing the housework and parenting skills with their respective spouses and children.

Unexpressed anger is one of the quickest ways to get cancer or a dis-ease of similar magnitude, in my opinion. If there is violence, there is no need for egotistic confrontation as the person is sick and has an emotional dis-ease. If you decide to leave, plan it quietly, do it gently, and do it quickly so as not to hurt or be hurt, and be secure and fair. Do not take what is not yours, or more than your half, rightfully earned, as you will not need that energy in your new life and truthfully you are better to start again, with none of the old energy if your life has been destructive. Build on a new wholesome energy that is nurturing and loving. IT IS NEVER TO LATE, AND YOU ARE NEVER TOO OLD TO START AGAIN. One of the greatest presidents in American history started about 100 times before successfully attaining the Presidency I am told so it is only ego and fear that hold us back from starting again.

Rape and child molestation, is wrong no matter how you feel about it, how much you love them, how sorry someone is about it, or what are the repercussions. A half-fulfilled life with fear is not a life that God wants you to live. **Report the situation**, the person is sick and needs help. You have not failed as you have a sick puppy on your hands and hopefully will get better after treatment/counseling. You will need counseling also. This is a positive step so you don't draw the same type of person into your life again if the relationship is irretrievable and will help you to understand we are not all the same nor have the same conditioning.

GET SUPPORT of friends/relatives or go to a shelter and get help. Take the risk of living, as everyone deserves to live well and happy, without idiots/bullies trying to control those weaker than they are by either violence or emotional blackmail. These bullies can be either male or female and will try everything in the book to avoid their little fantasy being known. The most common one is that no one must know or you will get worse but if you are not there and can't be found, that is a little hard to do. There are some wonderful people in the shelters now days whose job is to protect you and give you emotional support.

It is a universal law that if a person is a bully and preys on others then he must also be balanced with the whole spectrum by understanding what it is like to be bullied. Soul balancing its called. BULLIES HATE TO BE BULLIED.

YOUR BODY

Your home is your mental body so if your house is really untidy, usually you're mentally at your wit's end and may need to make some changes. It can be quite amazing that when you tidy up your home, other things seem to fall into place.

Your car is your emotional body and if your car has trouble starting it could mean that you have been lacking spark lately. Brakes failing may mean things are going too fast or you may need to put the brakes on. These signs can have positive or negative connotations. If your car is an old bomb and you are always having trouble then it's advisable to look at boosting your emotional body by doing something for you and trading in on a new automobile. The stronger the car or truck fourwheel drive the more dependable you will feel you are.

Your body is your self-image and so it seems to be divided into several sections.
- From the shoulders up to the top of the head is a thinking project. (Head crying syndrome/shoulders responsibility syndrome).
- Between the top of the shoulders to the top of the hips is what you are doing in your life.
- From the top of your hips to the tips of your toes is where you are going with your life. Your footsteps in life.

The body is further divided:
- The left side of the body is the female, creative, sensitive part of yourself.
- The right side of the body is the masculine, aggressive, strength, go ahead, get things done part of you.

When at times we keep knocking /hurting ourselves on specific areas of our bodies, interpretation may be made using the preceding formulae. These can be interpreted into the true way we are feeling in the subconscious mind and we can then change the pattern to avoid future pain. In an experiment a person was selected from passing people. He was bent over and looked for all intents and purposes like he was carrying the whole world on his shoulders. He was approached and told that he was to be given a large sum of money. Observers were quick to notice that he straightened up and looked proud and happy within a very short time. We have the same ability to turn the energy /electricity switch on within us and we can choose to wallow in our pain and suffering or change our internal switch like turning on the light in your own home.

All we have is now. God has not given us tomorrow. There is no guarantee in our back pocket that there is tomorrow. There is no guarantee at all. So if there is no tomorrow as it is not here, and maybe will never ever come, why worry about tomorrow? **All we have is now!** Yesterday is gone forever, and there is no use crying about it as it cannot be changed. There is no way possible in this time period to go back and change it even if we could, so let it go and ask yourself what did I learn from that experience? Maybe it was strength you learnt, maybe you will now, having had that experience, choose never to experience that again. Tuff luck WISDOM I call it.

Children have a wonderful ability to concentrate in the now and to fully enjoy all there is to offer. They have boundless mounds of energy as their mind's project into the moment..

As adults when we get to middle age we find that our memories are clouded about our childhood and seem to be ever fearful about the future. When this happens our minds are split three ways and so we become numb in our thinking. One third of our mind in the past with I should have, could have, regrets, etc. One third of our minds in the future, will I make it, will I have enough money to retire, will I have a house, will my kids be OK, etc. One third in the now. No wonder we are exhausted and feel like this life sucks!

Then when we get older and our bodies deteriorate and stiffen, we, who never had much of a memory at all about our past and childhood, suddenly can remember all the stories of our childhood and the fun we had. We don't want to keep our minds on our pains do we? We don't want to think about the future as there is not much time left and it is inevitable that we may die, so all of our mind energy looks into the past, which is also a belief.

Remember, if you can plan your day or week or year and then totally live in the now it is really amazing how all our aches and pains disappear as new life flows back into our bodies and minds. It is known among all therapists that the more clients concentrate on their obsession of their disease the more pain and growth it normally has.

Laughing at yourself can release so much tension, in fact there have been many people who have cured themselves of major diseases by getting funny DVD, video's and radio cassettes and laughing themselves to good health. Norman Cousins is well known in the USA as one of those people who cured himself of cancer by locking himself away in his room and laughed himself to good health. Omni magazine has stated in previous issues that hugs and shouting made bald men's hair grow and women's figures firm up. If you can't let go of your emotions as it may offend go for a drive and roll the windows up before you let rip, but be nice to your fellow drivers.

Close your bedroom door, tell everyone you do not want to be disturbed, grab a pillow, kneel by the bed and think of what is bothering you, and picture him/her/it on the pillow feeling your helplessness of the situation and take a deep breath. Bending over now with your arms under the pillow resting on the bed, but jammed against your mouth, yell and say all the things bugging you with force. The pillow and the bed will deaden the noise. By doing this at least three times you should feel spent but refreshed. Dr Craig Hassed of Monash University in Melbourne Australia has stated laughter reduces stress, improves mood and enhances a person's creativity. Stress increases levels of hormones ranging from adrenaline to cortisol, chemicals vital for the body in the right place and time. Out of balance they leave us open to illnesses. For example, high cortisol levels, linked to depression and chronic stress, are a risk factor for osteoporosis. Laughter eases stress and reduces levels of these potentially harmful hormones. Learn to laugh and it has been stated, to fake it is better than not laughing at all. Try to fake laughter for two minutes and you will really start to loosen up and genuine laughter at yourself will take place. Senior executives in the USA are being sent to laughter classes and do not be surprised if the next time you are in hospital wards and you see a Doctor with a clown nose on as children who are made to laugh are healing quicker.

LET GO OF THE DIS-EASE HOLDING YOU. LIVE FOR NOW!

DEATH AND DYING

Having had a death experience approximately 20 years ago and trying to understand my experience, I had the fortune to be able to talk to others who had a similar near death experience. We all agreed that it was one of the most freeing, beautiful experiences that we had ever had and to all intents and purposes death seemed to be like a passing through a veil into another dimension where the colors were much brighter and vibrant. A peace comes over you which is indescribable as the painful physical body drops away and ones soul/spirit leaves the body to be welcomed by their guidance or Guardian Angels. On one's orientation in the workings of the spiritual bodies these angels show the way back to where you are meant to be going for instruction as to whether it's your time to leave this planet or not.

Remember that you are a spark of God having the human experience, to return to God.

There is no separation from God unless using our free will deem it to be. When this happens dis-ease creeps in as we become out of balance.

I once had the fortune to be called to the presence of a holy man called Sai Baba in India, and he suggested that to pray outside of yourself to God separates one from oneself and allows other negative energies to manipulate your energies. Praying to God within your own temple will go direct as we are built from the spark of The Great Mystery's image. Remember also that when you get angry, condemn yourself, criticize yourself then you are also criticizing and saying GOD is no good too. Not a good policy as it may give the answers or the attention you are not looking or praying for.

I have heard from so many people who have been deathly afraid of an operation say after the near death experience (N.D.E.) and the operation that their lives were so busy and they obviously were not listening.
This was the time that their guidance gave them a fine-tuning while their bodies were being operated on. They somehow felt different after the operation on a deep level of their being and their life was different with less worry and stress. Death was no longer a fear. Having had this near death experience we all agreed that if God called and said for us to go home now we would say our goodbyes if there was time enough and leave happily.
Most people afterwards said that their gifts were heightened and they could quite often see the things that go bump in the night that others did not see and understand. Their clairvoyant gifts improved. On attending funerals of friends, clairvoyants will tell you that quite often they will sense the friend sitting on the coffin or around the family looking very bewildered. After explanation in the mind as to what is happening to them and what would be best for them to do, they are usually quite happy to go into the light and leave and go home. At this point however it is important to state that it is not in the highest interest of any recently deceased soul to be kept earthbound, because we who are left don't want them to leave.

Too often I have seen a persons manifest the same disease as their loved one died from by holding on. On releasing the soul the symptom of dis-ease left almost immediately like in a miracle. The films Ghost and Always are good examples of what happens after death and have obviously been written by people who have either had a near death experience or have done their homework on the subject.

THE IMMUNE SYSTEM

This system is the most underrated system in the human body and its importance is too often overlooked.

The immune system is like the fixer upper of our plumbing system, acting as grease trap, waste dump and helping and working in conjunction with the lymphatic system in energetic form. It also enables the carriers of energy and food to all of the body and mind to do their jobs with clarity and integrity. It's responsibility is to remove out of the system all of the waste products that are too acid to excrete and can cause us harm. If the body did excrete too much acidic waste from the system, there would be large liver /kidney /bladder and reproductory infections as our delicate vessels would not be able to cope with this, and we would end up with horrid sores appearing inside the tubing, all over our sensitive areas.

Have you ever had strong soap inside sensitive areas? If you have you will know what I mean as it feels like barbed wire been drawn through the tube. If our immune system gets too stressed and the lymphatic system can't cope, it dumps acidic and toxic fluid into and between our joints eventually causing stiffness. The immune system acts like the local council dumping rubbish at the designated dumps of tissue or in between joints. If this condition is really bad in our bodies joints become stiff, tissues become inflamed and burn like an acid is on them and is labelled arthritis.

It also seems that if toxicity level gets too high then it comes out to the skin level and causes pimples, rashes, and boils to get this damaging toxicity out of the system. One of the worst problems that the immune system has to face seems to be a toxic colon, where years of wrong eating, not taking care, and not enough exercise has finally caught up with us. It does not stop there! Antibiotics, childhood diseases like mumps, measles, inoculations with some live vaccines, strep infections, croup, etc. and also amalgam fillings containing mercury all have an effect of slowing the immune system's efficiency down so we end up feeling like death warmed up.

What changes can we implement to improve the immune system?

Water

Get a filter for your water system and drink the required eight glasses of fresh water every day even though you may feel a little waterlogged for a while. As a matter of interest regarding the cleanliness of water, I was sponsored to teach a weekend class in Colorado on self-healing a few years ago. During the class I made an announcement as it came from my guides or guardian angels to warn the class not to drink the water, and if this was not possible, at least boil it or buy water in plastic bottles from another state. There was still a risk there of plastic contamination. When a low-grade plastic gets hot then cools down rapidly, it can put a form of formaldehyde in the water that is bad for the immune system. I think they thought I was a bit of a crank or an alarmist until the following day there was a story in the local newspaper that the local water supply was contaminated by nerve gas which had been buried after the war effort. Some of the steel barrels had rusted through and leaked into the water table and people had been taken to hospital in a very bad way.

COPY OF NEWS IN DENVER POST FOLLOWS

THURSDAY

Warm Late Storms
High 85-87

THE DENVER POST

uly 26, 1990 · · · · · · · · · · · · · · · *Voice of the Rocky Mountain Empire* · · · · · · · · · · · · · · · Final Edition / 25 cents

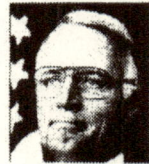

INSIDE THE POST

Nerve-gas byproduct taints water

71 families warned not to use their wells

By Steve Lipsher
Denver Post Staff Writer

The Colorado Health Department today is warning 71 Adams County families not to drink or cook with their well water, which tests reveal has been tainted with a nerve-gas byproduct from the Rocky Mountain Arsenal.

Results of a department study of 121 sites released yesterday show that a chemical called DIMP or diisopropylmethylphosphonate disposed of by the Army on the arsenal from the 1950s to the 1970s, has migrated underground north and northwest into water supplies.

"As a precaution, we have advised 71 of the families not to drink or cook with their domestic well water, since DIMP was detected in their wells," said Dr. Tom Vernon, health department executive director.

Chloroform also was detected in eight of the 11 locations, which included residences and businesses, Vernon said last night.

The health department and the Environmental Protection Agency have agreed to pay for bottled water for the people affected for as much as three to four years. That would cost about $50,000 a year, said Jeff Edson, who is overseeing the arsenal cleanup for the health department.

The 27-square-mile arsenal, an EPA Superfund cleanup site, has been called one of the most contaminated sites on Earth.

For decades, the U.S. government produced nerve gases at the arsenal. Shell Oil Co. produced and tested pesticides there, as well.

DIMP was detected in levels ranging from 6.1 parts per billion to 148 parts per billion, Edson said.

The EPA has established 600 parts per billion as the maximum acceptable level of DIMP in water, but the state health department has not set standards.

Please see ARSENAL *on 12A*

Many councils have saved money by laying asbestos pipes down to bring water to you and these give off small fibres of asbestos which in turn has been connected to stomach cancer, so water needs to be filtered.

Filter your showers too!

Chlorine added to most municipal water supplies, is a disinfectant that hardens arteries, destroys proteins in the body, irritates skin and sinus conditions, and aggravates asthma, allergies and respiratory problems.

Chloroform: By-product of chlorination causes excessive free radical formation (accelerated aging) normal cells to mutate, and cholesterol to oxidise. It is a known carcinogen, producing cancer in the body.

DCA (Dichloro acedic acid): Chlorine by-product alters cholesterol metabolism and has been shown to cause liver cancer in lab animals.

MX (another chlorinated acid: By-product of chlorination, MX is known to cause genetic mutations that can lead to cancer growth and has been found in all chlorinated water for which it was tested.

It's a proven cause of bladder and rectal cancer. Research at Harvard University and the Medical College of Wisconsin has proven that chlorinated water is the direct cause of 9 per cent of all bladder cancers and 15 per cent of all rectal cancers in the USA

Evidence is there that chlorine destroys protein in your body. This disinfectant bleach makes your hair and scalp dry, worsens dandruff, ruins chemically treated hair and can make these conditions worse, asthma and sinus conditions, allergies, skin rashes, emphysema.

Your body can absorb more chlorine in a 10 minute shower than if you drank eight glasses of the same water as a warm shower opens up your pores.

As a result you inhale the chlorine vapours directly through the skin, also directly into the bloodstream. A risk a day will not keep the doctor away

The answer is clear. Stop chlorinating your body and get a good filter!

There is a researcher in Japan who has taken samples of water in many special places in the world frozen them and taken photos of them. The crystalline effects are really beautiful and have to been seen to believed. For example what is interesting is that in an oil filled water lake the samples crystalline effect is really muddy and no reflective energy compared to those samples taken at Lourdes or blessed water from a church which really sparkled.

The same goes on a water sample taken from a house where there has been arguments and one where there is much love and respect for each other.

If we are made up of 95 per cent water it also means to me that it is important for us to be in or choose to be in a loving environment to have health and happiness!

Environment

In Australia there have been cases of radioactive sand being buried or treated improperly and some families in State housing have ended up with strange sores on children's legs and arms. A few serious cancerous diseases of the blood are also showing up because not enough care has been taken to neutralize or dispose of the waste material properly.

You must remember that to get rid of this kind of waste properly costs millions of dollars and to pay someone to give them the go ahead to use this type of material may be a lot cheaper if you don't have a conscience. Unscrupulous companies have millions of dollars worth of insurance to cover any complaint. If they stall your complaint for a few years you may be dead, so it won't cost them anything much. Maybe the evidence is then buried. Sad but true.

There is recent evidence obtained that the nuclear power plants are not at all safe either. I have been told that since Chernobyl many people are falling ill from eating the radioactive fish caught in the northern hemisphere and in the Pacific area after the French nuclear testing in French Polynesia. Sickening! If you don't believe me then talk to Greenpeace and support them in protecting our environment.

On doing a scan with the Se-5 Intrinsic Data field Analyzer which analyses and works on the Scalar waves for a very sick friend and client in an north eastern state of the USA, I was amazed to find that she had radioactivity in her immune system as well as all the chemicals usually associated with a nuclear explosion. Before balancing her out after doing the scan I asked whether there was any form of nuclear activity going on around her, to which she replied there was a nuclear submarine base a short distance away and an old nuclear power plant only 20 miles away. I asked if she had heard about a spill and she had not so I informed her to take many things to boost her immune system as the scan showed there had been a spill.

A couple of days later she phoned and informed me that the papers had reported a small spill had occurred. I informed her that from the instrumentation I had, the size of the spill was worse than what they had told the public. She should keep boosting her immune system as much as possible and suggested she leave the area as soon as possible as there will be a lot of people getting sick from the damage done to the immune systems from radioactive overloading.

One month later she phoned me to say hundreds of local people had very strange virus problems. They had found out that approximately 50 guys who worked at the station had sat on a chair where a minor spill had happened at the station and have or are being tested for testicle cancer or similar. The authorities are now thinking of giving the public in the State some pills to boost the immune system just in case an emergency comes up.

SCARY TO THINK THESE PEOPLE IN CHARGE OF THESE PROJECTS CAN GET AWAY WITH SUCH BLATANT IRRESPONSIBLE-LIFE THREATENING BEHAVIOUR ISNT IT?
To be forewarned is to be forearmed and let me assure you that with so many greedy people in charge of this world it is not going to get any better. Buy the best pure water filter and house water filtration system you can buy as soon as possible if you value quality of life. You can't live without good water and there are many reports on the Internet stating that most of the diseases we have are caused by the body's dehydration and not drinking enough water.

Essiac Tea /Flor-Essence Tea

If you do have cancer then make enquires about the Essiac tea that is a blend of herbs formulated from an well-known Ojebwe Indian formula. Rene Caisse, a nurse in Canada, administered and had incredible success of reducing the effects of terminal cancer in-patients and in some cases went into remission. There are glowing reports from patients on http://www.herbalhealer.com

The Health Sciences Institute in the USA has an advisory council consisting of many physicians and other health professionals. These experts offer new revolutionary treatments from all over the world in cutting edge cancer cures for cancer from the Amazon rainforest to Australian outback asthma breakthroughs and where you can obtain the products. (www.HSIBaltimore.com)

Coffee /Ginseng Tea

If you are like me you love your organic coffee! I know it can give us constipation, make us hyper and have complications but the smell and taste is so good isn't it?

Organic coffee is blended from 100 per cent coffee beans and the flavour is a lot better. No artificial chemicals and natural methods of cultivation make this coffee a little more expensive, but oh so good! (www.clipper-teas.com)

Suggest instead of overdosing on coffee you limit the coffee to one to two cups a day and purchase some Korean ginseng tea and have it with water twice daily. It's a great pick-me-up and good for you too! And so is a glass of hot water with the juice of a half of lemon, or herbal tea first thing in the morning as it starts your colon and bowel moving.

Food

Watch what you eat and purchase and buy organic fruit and vegetables wherever possible. Make sure your vegetables are washed well in filtered water and cooked to stop parasite infestation. Preferably steamed in filtered water. You might be saying that this is not possible but according to some scientists there is a parasitical high at the moment so you can't be too careful. In 1996 a meeting of all the leading parasitologists was called in Tucson, Arizona to discuss the high incidence in hospitals of the increase of parasites affecting patients' health and what were the best cures. In some countries parasites are so bad that there is virtually nothing the doctors can do.

(Buy a Zapper and read A Cure For All Diseases by Hulda Clarke)

Find out what you are allergic to in food lines and avoid these as much as possible. Eat live food wherever possible, avoid moldy foods and cook using as little oil and grease as possible.

High-speed convection oven and a steamer are great, and inexpensive. Use a little butter and cold pressed virgin olive oil as some of the latest research denigrates some of the cooking oils, and aerosol cans of oil and margarine. Until I have researched them I will stay with what I know.

Wherever possible avoid dairy foods, cheese, milk, etc. especially if you have allergies or sinus problems. Use organic dairy if you really cannot do without milk. Leave the soy alone.

Raw foods and wok cooking seem good and healthy. You do not see too many overweight Japanese and Chinese people unless they want to be a Sumo wrestler or something similar.

Read labels on food and find out what they mean and what they do. A good friend of mine once said if you couldn't pronounce it don't have it.

Have a read of some of the things that go into ice-cream.

MOST ICE-CREAM IS SYNTHETIC THESE DAYS:

LOS ANGELES - A school custodian observed that spilled ice-cream sometimes hardens and refuses to be washed off with water it was reported there. Perhaps, the report continued, content of the cream had some thing to do with it.

Modern ice-cream, it went on, is fantastically synthetic now, and contains:

DIGITAL GLYCOL an emulsifier used in place of eggs, and also used in antifreeze and paint remover.

PIPERONAL	is used instead of vanilla and also used to kill lice.
ALDEHYDE C17	cherry flavor, an inflammable liquid used in dyes, plastics, and rubber.
ETHYL ACETATE	for pineapple flavour, BUTRALDEHYDE as nut flavour, AMYL as banana flavor and BENZYL ACETATE for strawberry flavor are not only used in ice-cream but are also used in cleaning fluids, rubber cement, oil paint solvent and nitrate solvent.

From **Organic Seeds For Thot**

And we wonder why nations of people are sick and depressed.

Water or soft drinks similar to Coke

75 per cent of the people are chronically deficient/dehydrated in water, which means our bodies are not sufficiently hydrated, and this being the case toxins are not flushed out of our bodies.

We then resort to soft drinks/pop drinks designed to have sugar in them to make us drink more.

Synthetic/Chemical Sugar /Neurotoxins /MSG

Aspartame/Nutrasweet/Equal/Spoonful etc. Most of these sweeties have connections to multiple sclerosis, systemic lupus, fibromyalgia spasms, shooting pains, numbness, cramps, memory loss and many more anomalies. Think you will lose weight by taking them? I have read that to think of these chemical sweetners as a minute nerve gas that could eliminate brain and nerve function and Aspartame makes you crave carbohydrates and you gain weight. The formaldehyde stores on the hips and thighs.

After reading on the Internet that someone was repackaging and selling it as ant poison I personally killed several ant nests by sprinkling one of these products around an ant nest to check the validity of the statement. Imagine my amazement when two days later the ants were gone! Watch what you put in your mouth!

One good way to kick start your body all over again and wash a lot of toxins out of the system is to have a series of colonics.

Colon Therapy

Find a professional, certified colon therapist who is recommended by Doctors of Homeopathy or Naturopathy and have a series of colonic irrigations. When I say this most people make all the excuses under the sun to avoid it, and even suggest that they will take chemicals and herbs to do the job instead. They usually come back a couple of months later looking and feeling exactly the same. They use excuses like I am embarrassed, it might hurt, and I might mess up. I once used those excuses too, and am now really grateful and have for the last 10 years had a series of three very close together at least once a year.

Warm controlled water is fed into your colon and the stomach is massaged. When the stomach becomes uncomfortable it is vacuumed out so there is very little mess. You can even carry on a conversation while doing this. A professional person is also available if a particularly hard blockage needs to be broken up using massage before being extracted. You can do this therapy yourself but to me it is very messy and very time consuming and you need someone on hand to help you if you get stuck.

If you do this yourself you need to make or purchase from the local drug store a Colonic bottle with a long tube and a flow control to be able to shut the water off when needed, and an insertion plug. Get the instructions. Filtered warm water needs to be gravitationally fed into the anal canal using a new inserter every time. Insist on this every time with a professional person doing this job. Warm water flows up towards the stomach while you lay on your back or side on a table (in an empty bath at home is suggested for the do it yourselfer) with a maximum amount of two to three pints of water in the water bottle. This excretion water needs to be expressed into the toilet every time the pressure buildup becomes intolerable and it is necessary to massage the stomach and intestine area to break up the lumps. As you need to do this at least three times every morning and night for at least seven days to get the maximum water penetration in the intestines, it may be cheaper, requires lots of patience but, can sometimes be embarrassing.

John Chamberlin

If you want to do this yourself, buy a recommended book on how to do it for yourself first or talk to someone who personally does it this way, and looks happy and vibrant and full of energy.

Suggested three books are;
Tissue Cleansing Through Bowel Management By Bernard Jensen.
Colon Health: The Key to a Vibrant Life by Norman Walker and
The Colon Health Handbook by Robert Gray

Eating wrong foods similar to simulated cheese, which as you know tastes and looks like liquid plastic and can be found piled on a hamburger at nameless fast food places, gets caught up in the little pulps or little bulb shaped tissue which hangs down in the intestine tubes. Simply put, the pulps job is meant to catch all the vitamins and minerals that our bodies need. Then its job is to transmute the good food value over to the bloodstream to where it is transported to the rest of the cells and the body to give us energy and good health. What happens normally however is that our intestines have ended up like a rusty pipe. It doesn't matter what food value we eat, what vitamins/ minerals we take, if your colon is rusty or clogged it's hard to get the vitamins/minerals value out of food as most of it goes to the sewer because it cannot be processed through the walls of the intestine.

When the colon becomes constipated generally it is packed or lined with accumulated, hardened faeces lodged in the pockets of the colon walls. This can happen after taking doses of antibiotics which kill off not only the viruses but also the good bacteria we need for assimilation. This hardened matter then obstructs the muscular contractions (peristalsis waves) and more faeces build-up along the walls resulting in the colon's inability to properly evacuate. Waste build-up of many years can actually result in up to 15 pounds of extra weight causing a distended and abnormally shaped colon and normally an overhung extended stomach. The clogged colon then interferes with final absorption and digestion of food, depriving the body of necessary nutrients. The results of this are fermentation and putrefaction of undigested food which carries poison that is

138

reabsorbed into the body and bloodstream and carried to every part of the body causing tired and listless feelings. The brain and nervous system become depressed and irritable, the lungs can create a foul breath and stressful breathing. Also the digestive organs create skin problems and sallow complexion with joints becoming stiff and painful due to toxic deposits.

If your colon is not in good healthy order you will end up with the most expensive sewer around as even the most expensive vitamin/minerals that you take and all the goodness of nutritious food is going to end up there. It is really important to get lots of fiber in your diet as it is really common practice now for westerners to have thickened walls in the colon causing constant pain because we eat too many refined foods.

A HEALTHY COLON IS YOUR HEALTH. I do not understand why so many doctors are so against colonic irrigation. Probably because sometimes this process does cause some pain and in the old primitive days some infections used to arise but with modern sterilized equipment this is very seldom. Colonic therapy is one of the first things given to diseased patients in most of the leading health resorts of renown centers like the Edgar Casey Center in Phoenix USA dealing with terminally ill patients. Some of these patients have up to 12 visits to the colon therapist in twelve days. One patient had complained of stomach pains all her life to find on the twelfth Colonic a small marble dropped out. She has not had the same pain in her stomach since and on investigation from her parents found out that the marble was swallowed at something like three years of age.

I am only asking you after being checked out by a Homeopathic or Naturopathic Doctor, to have a series of three Colonics over three days. Why three days did I hear you ask? The first of these, especially if you have never had one, never seems to clean you out and the water doesn't go all the way. The second one will go all the way and the third one will make sure you are squeaky clean. How do we avoid all this in the future?

- Drink lots of clean fresh filtered water. Eight glasses a day is the required minimum for a healthy colon and for the intestine to be kept moist and regular. Avoid coffee where possible if you have a constipation problem as it does, among other things, bind you up... but enough about coffee, I like it too.
- Have fiber in your breakfast cereal, but get kinesiology or SE-5 Intrinsic Data Field Analyzer tested for what food energy suits your system and is allergy free for you. Some people have bad reactions to wheat bran for instance, and could be taking rice bran instead as an alternative.
- Take acidophilus/bifidus three times a day, or at least twice a day for at least seven days before you have your series of colonics. That will put the right acid/alkaline balance into your stomach, thereby helping the right flora to gain enough strength to keep the disease causing bacteria at bay. Primadophilus in the refrigerated form and the refrigerated Blackmore's brand are also giving very good results. Continue this for a least one to two months afterwards. Our colon and intestine is similar to a septic tank and has to have the right bug and acid/alkaline balance to give good service. Remember, as said before, an unbalanced colon can in energy form cause heartburn, acidity, ulcers, shortness of breath, bad and putrefied breath, and a lot of excess weight by putting water in the tissues when the liver and kidneys cannot process all the toxicity. If this is the case, the urine is too toxic and maybe acidic, the bladder cannot cope without getting infection and can't pee it out, and the subconscious mind will put it into the fat or muscle tissues instead. Dry faeces blocked in the colon behind the bladder area causing pressure on the bladder and or the prostate has also been known to cause imbalances. Colonics are a great help in balancing Candida Albicans, in conjunction with diet and the right herbs.

I cannot stress the importance strongly enough of getting your colon cleaned if medically possible, if you have any type of dis-ease.

If you wish to go the medical route and you have been diagnosed ulcers, then check for the detection of helicobacter pylori (Urea breath test) as there have been many people cured after this treatment who thought they were incurable. Quick Cleanse Intestinal Cleansing Program is a herbal intestinal broom is also a good product for the wimps who won't do the colonic program.

Candida Albicans

This affects probably one out of three of people's systems and needs to be treated. Candida Albicans looks like an alga in the ocean. It settles in the mucosal surface of the intestine and will not bother us when kept in check. It is a simple yeast fungus that grows on the surface of nearly every living thing and also thrives in the bodies of most animals and humans. Candida Albicans poses no threat when its population in the body is held at normal levels. In days gone by children got thrush in the mouth. People had trouble with depression, athlete's foot, fungus infection of the nails, or jock itch. Some were made worse when exposed to perfumes, tobacco smoke, and other chemicals, on damp days or working in moldy places.

The natural friendly bacteria combatants of Candida Albicans, the active good bacteria usually counteracted these problems quickly in a healthy person. Leading immunologists estimate that 80 million Americans (one out of every three) are already suffering from Candida Albicans. When diagnosed with Candida Albicans there is an abnormally high level of fungus in the intestinal tract and it reaches the fatal stage when toxins enter the bloodstream and start biting the hypothalamus causing all types of mental aberrations from suicidal depression to homicidal attacks.

This is toxic brain poisoning, not an emotional problem and not everyone's system is the same. The waste of the fungus attacks the nervous system. Since the advent of penicillin or derivatives being put in cattle food and chicken mash etc. it comes to our table and along with modern drugs like birth control pills, steroids, and broad spectrum antibiotics, a lot of the good lactobacillus is killed off giving symptoms of;
- Frequent headaches
- Yeast infections
- Dizziness

- Blurred vision
- Poor digestion
- Rectal itch
- Fatigue
- Rashes
- Nausea
- White coating on the tongue
- Allergies of most types

Advanced symptoms can be;
- Sensitivity to moulds
- Gastritis
- Bloating
- Constipation
- Diarrhea
- Gas colitis
- Headaches
- Lethargy
- Fatigue
- Hives
- Food allergies
- Chemical sensitivities
- Hyperactivity
- Acne
- Yeast vaginitis
- Menstrual irregularities
- Cramping
- Kidney and bladder infections
- Cystitis
- Allergic symptoms like hay fever/sinusitis
- Earache
- Cold hands and feet
- Joint pains that travel from place to place
- Numbness

See your Homeopathic Doctor or make an appointment at the A.R.E. Clinic at 4018 North 40 th Street Phoenix AZ 85018 Phone 602-955-0551 where if applicable to your case they will give you Nystatin or Nysoral to control Candida Albicans.

If you think some of these symptoms are yours, write to Kroeger Herbs 1122 Pearl Street, Boulder, CO 80302 Phone 303-443-0261 for her herbal mixture.

Get a yeast free diet program from your doctor. Watch your diet as it will have to be free of yeast products and anything that ferments like wine, beer, malts, mushrooms, cheeses, vinegar, dried fruits and melons, especially cantaloupe. Other foods to avoid are also peanuts because of the mould, cakes, candies, ice-cream, soft drinks, honey, maple syrup, carob and any sugar as cancer feeds on sugar containing foods. Feels like you throat has been cut for a while but when your energy levels improve the diet can be relaxed a little.

Back/Spine Health

Go to a chiropractor, or a naturopath who is certified to massage and manipulate your back and spine as the vertebrae in your spine can, if out of alignment, cause all sorts of pains including phantom pains, in areas that are not in actually in trouble. Preferably go to a practitioner who will take the time and massage use heat and relax your muscles /ligaments first.

What happens to a pinched nerve is similar to this. When you take a garden hose, turn on the water and start to spray the garden with water, and if someone comes up behind you and puts a crimp in the hose, the water flow slows down or stops doesn't it? The same thing happens when our negative thinking affects us or the vertebrae are out of alignment. When you are straining and working too hard physically or mentally, the subconscious mind pulls the spine out of alignment. When this happens, it's like the hose on diminished power flow, as the vertebrae put increased pressure on the nerves that run between them. This cuts off the nerve message input and output to the brain and organ it represents. Thus the messages to and from the brain are confused. Let's say the back is painful and out of alignment between the 3 rd, 4 th and 5 th lumbar. This will mean that the message is carried to the brain that there is a problem at the corresponding nerve endings and to balance or fix the problem by compensating. On assessing the situation the subconscious mind may even send extra hormones etc. there to the sex organs, uterus, bladder or prostate gland which are not needed. It may unnecessarily compensate in the muscular system which could put extra pressure on the 5 th lumbar causing sciatic nerve problems that can often cause a person to end up in bed for long spells with paralysed legs and knees.

A good suggestion if you continue to have projects with your back and joints is to take Emu oil internally in tablet form and also topically on the joints. Added supplements that work to help are Shark cartilage 1000mg to rebuild the cartilage and get rid of small parasites in the tissues as a side effect.

Glucosamine Sulfate 1000mg to help the ligaments and Natural fish oil 1000mg or Flax oil which has all the Omega 3,6, and 9 fatty acids to help the joints in prevention of arthritis and help with peripheral circulation. This helped the old man in me taking a long time to get out of the bed in the morning back to getting straight up without pain.

Emu oil or Goanna Joint Eze Oil applied topically every night and morning helped immensely.

Emu oil has been used by the Aboriginals for centuries for its anti-inflammatory and arthritic conditions and Emu Omega 369 has reportedly been found to be beneficial in chronic fatigue, migraines, asthma and a host of other ailments. (www.emuspirit.com)

Tai Chi is known in China for centuries to be effective in relieving arthritis and is a gentle and effective relaxing exercise program as is **Yoga** in India. Both are excellent and several videos are now available to do in the privacy in your own home until you feel supple enough to going to a class. (www.taichiproductions.com)

Babies

Babies from about seven days old who have colic (digestive upsets /can't hold food down) respond really well to your favourite chiropractor /osteopath realigning the back behind the stomach and shoulders using his thumbs. What has usually happened is no fault of the midwife/doctor but if a little arm/leg has been pulled too hard during birthing then the little backs get pulled out of alignment. This in turn causes pain stress on the nerves going into the stomach /chest etc. I believe it is imperative that all baby's should be checked out by a chiropractor /osteopath within the first 10 days of birth to stop the incredible pain the little ones have to go through in our ignorance. I have experienced where a chiropractor worked on the mother as her back was out of alignment to put the babies back in alignment. The baby obviously was an inpath and was in sympathy with the energy. Unless the back / neck is critical no X-rays please. He should be able to do this from his experience.

If the baby cries a lot for no apparent reason, you have checked its diet, is in warm dry non itchy clothing, is clean, cuddled and held, has had reassuring skin touch, and had its back put in, the flowers taken out of the room, kicked the cat, dog or birds out, have anti-allergy bedding to stop dust mites etc.

Then move the crib a few feet from where it is as its bed could be on a Hartmann line. Dr Hartmann has proof after working on thousands of people that this theory works and believes that there could be a correlation to Hartmann lines and cot deaths. More later about Hartmann lines.

COPY OF PARKER CHIROPRACTIC RESEARCH
FOUNDATION SPINE CHART
FOLLOWS

Look at the correlation of what mixed signals causes pressure on nerves in the spine and how you are affected.

CHART OF EFFECTS OF SPINAL MISALIGNMENTS

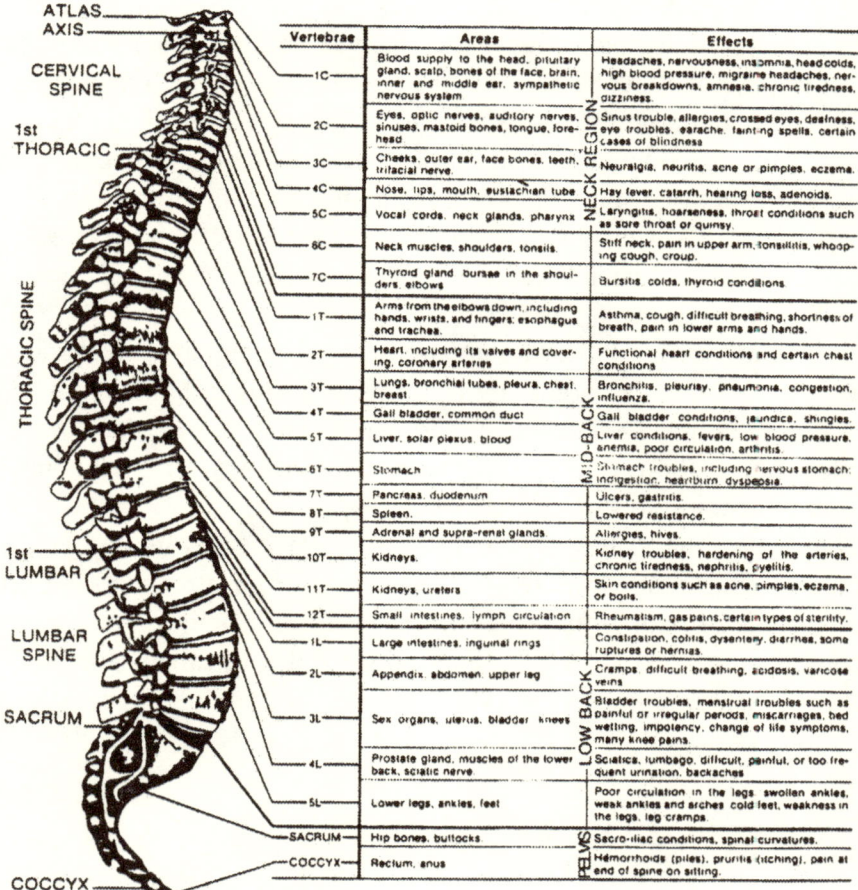

Vertebrae	Areas	Effects
1C	Blood supply to the head, pituitary gland, scalp, bones of the face, brain, inner and middle ear, sympathetic nervous system	Headaches, nervousness, insomnia, head colds, high blood pressure, migraine headaches, nervous breakdowns, amnesia, chronic tiredness, dizziness.
2C	Eyes, optic nerves, auditory nerves, sinuses, mastoid bones, tongue, forehead	Sinus trouble, allergies, crossed eyes, deafness, eye troubles, earache, fainting spells, certain cases of blindness
3C	Cheeks, outer ear, face bones, teeth, trifacial nerve.	Neuralgia, neuritis, acne or pimples, eczema.
4C	Nose, lips, mouth, eustachian tube	Hay fever, catarrh, hearing loss, adenoids.
5C	Vocal cords, neck glands, pharynx	Laryngitis, hoarseness, throat conditions such as sore throat or quinsy.
6C	Neck muscles, shoulders, tonsils.	Stiff neck, pain in upper arm, tonsillitis, whooping cough, croup.
7C	Thyroid gland, bursae in the shoulders, elbows	Bursitis, colds, thyroid conditions.
1T	Arms from the elbows down, including hands, wrists, and fingers; esophagus and trachea	Asthma, cough, difficult breathing, shortness of breath, pain in lower arms and hands.
2T	Heart, including its valves and covering, coronary arteries	Functional heart conditions and certain chest conditions
3T	Lungs, bronchial tubes, pleura, chest, breast	Bronchitis, pleurisy, pneumonia, congestion, influenza.
4T	Gall bladder, common duct	Gall bladder conditions, jaundice, shingles.
5T	Liver, solar plexus, blood	Liver conditions, fevers, low blood pressure, anemia, poor circulation, arthritis.
6T	Stomach	Stomach troubles, including nervous stomach; indigestion, heartburn, dyspepsia.
7T	Pancreas, duodenum	Ulcers, gastritis.
8T	Spleen.	Lowered resistance.
9T	Adrenal and supra-renal glands.	Allergies, hives.
10T	Kidneys.	Kidney troubles, hardening of the arteries, chronic tiredness, nephritis, pyelitis.
11T	Kidneys, ureters	Skin conditions such as acne, pimples, eczema, or boils.
12T	Small intestines, lymph circulation	Rheumatism, gas pains, certain types of sterility.
1L	Large intestines, inguinal rings	Constipation, colitis, dysentery, diarrhea, some ruptures or hernias.
2L	Appendix, abdomen, upper leg	Cramps, difficult breathing, acidosis, varicose veins
3L	Sex organs, uterus, bladder, knees	Bladder troubles, menstrual troubles such as painful or irregular periods, miscarriages, bed wetting, impotency, change of life symptoms, many knee pains.
4L	Prostate gland, muscles of the lower back, sciatic nerve.	Sciatica, lumbago, difficult, painful, or too frequent urination, backaches.
5L	Lower legs, ankles, feet.	Poor circulation in the legs, swollen ankles, weak ankles and arches, cold feet, weakness in the legs, leg cramps.
SACRUM	Hip bones, buttocks	Sacro-iliac conditions, spinal curvatures.
COCCYX	Rectum, anus	Hemorrhoids (piles), pruritis (itching), pain at end of spine on sitting.

Misalignments of spinal vertebrae and discs may cause irritation to the nervous system and affect the structures, organs, and functions which may result in the conditions shown above.

Teeth / Mouth Hygiene

If not looked after teeth can make you depressed and there have been many cases of people going crazy when the toxins from decaying teeth went into the brain.

In acupuncture your teeth are attached through the meridians to different parts of the body so it could mean that that pesky tooth could be causing the phantom pain in the stomach. Definitely if the tooth filling of Amalgam is cracked and leaking.

Ulcers are a sure sign that your dental hygiene is not up to scratch and I have found Cepacol from the normal drug store to be one of the best for an ulcerated mouth and has been known to kill a raw nerve. Colloidal silver is more natural but a little slower. Oraced tincture of cloves is for a tooth that is hurting but mind your tongue as it will numb it too if you touch it. It comes in a Jelly for young childrens gums too.

If you have a lot of depression or pain go and see your friendly dentist and get your tooth fixed as a infected mouth is a ticking time bomb and in my own experience has a habit of giving trouble just when you least want or need it. Amalgams, which is the filler used to fill teeth in bygone days have a low-level mercury in them and many other toxic chemicals. Have your dentist give you a quote on extracting the amalgams and replacing it with the new white materials now available. Biocalex has been used in Europe for years successfully.

My own experience in this was really astonishing and gave me a flatter stomach, less throat problems and much more energy and brain vitality.

Keep your teeth cleaned at least twice a day to keep plaque and bacteria at bay.

If you can't afford toothpaste then use filtered water and also several old remedies like salt and Bi-Carb of soda but not too much salt or you will damage the enamel. Pure water is as good as any. Avoid toothpastes with sodium laurel sulfate (SLS), a detergent foam that is listed as a primary irritant and a poison in the USA. This product is also used in hair shampoos, cosmetics, baby bath etc. Some toothpaste have chlorhexidren, bromchlorophen and even formaldehyde as antibacterials. The stripe toothpaste dyes in some can be absorbed through the gums into the body really quickly too. When buying, purchase organic toothpaste!

Vitamins and Minerals

We already have in our bodies all the vitamins, minerals, herbal potions and lotions that our bodies ever need. All we have to do is harness our subconscious mind and brain to supply them or at least attract us to the food with these vitamins etc., in to alleviate any imbalanced situation.

When my children were young and they had a headache or sore tummy we used to make up a bread pill and tell them it would fix the headache if they took it with a glass of water. This pain condition was monitored but in 95 per cent of the cases the child would report the pain gone in a very short time.

This is called a placebo and these pills are still manufactured today in all different colours and yes, you still pay for them. We as humans are so conditioned to take a pill to fix up a problem that if you imagine taking a vitamin / mineral /painkiller /to relax the muscle, etc. when no drugs are available the subconscious mind will send various chemicals and relax the area that is in the pain area to fix the problem. This does work with practice and can be confirmed by any hypnotherapist.

What the mind believes is achieved. It's like having a Clayton's non alcoholic drink, a drink when you are not having a drink. Clayton's health? A Pill when you are not having a pill.

If you are not able to condition your mind into believing this at this time then go to a naturopath or similar and get them to test you for the vitamins/minerals that are compatible for your body. It is normal for you to be unique and not fall into everyone else's category. Everyone can take vitamin C and vitamin B. Right? Wrong!

For years I could not understand that if I took vitamin B or C why I felt really sick shortly after and was told by those who are meant to know that the more I took the more my body would accept it. I did tell you I used to be very gullible didn't I.

Find a therapist who knows how to find out how your body reacts to different chemicals, vitamins, minerals and checks by using kinesiology. I know is not foolproof but it is a lot better than a guessing game. Failing that, be in touch with the writer or publisher of this book and names can be sent of a local SE-5 practitioner who can test your body for what your body wants and needs for health. This test is determined from either a hair sample, blood sample or a Polaroid photograph sample. During a personal session the SE-5 can also tell off samples of the vitamin/mineral if the brands that you have bought are really compatible with your system or not.

It is not necessary in my opinion to be taking wads and wads of supplements, as some will have us believe. When you take them, how you take them and what others pills/vitamins you take with them is also crucial as some vitamins and minerals mixed together can cause immediate stress to the body. Excessive chemicals, herbs etc. can cause chronic fatigue and can make your dis-ease even worse because the immune system is battling a chemical swamp inside your stomach and system.

I met a lady in Arizona who had been diagnosed with chronic fatigue and when I did a healing her whole body felt like chemical soup so I asked her when she made her next appointment to bring in all the supplements she had with her. Boy was I surprised when she arrived up with a suitcase of them. Out of 34 bottles of all these vitamin/ mineral supplements, we found that she not only didn't need 29 of them but also the way she was taking them was disastrous and her stomach and immune system was like a chemical soup. She had been listening to all the so called experts and well meaning friends who said this worked for them, and bought whatever everyone suggested in the desperation to be well. Been there, done that.
The nice ending to the story was that she learnt to discriminate/ discern and only took the three or four vitamins /minerals suggested and was back to work in a few weeks with a much-renewed energy.

It is important to give your body a well-deserved rest at least once a year and take no supplements for a least a month. Medical drugs too need resting if your doctor let's you and if it does not cause too much stress to you. Let the body and mind realign itself chemically

/energy wise. Then retest yourself and you may find you do not need them as much as you needed them before.

From body testing and using the SE-5 testing in the USA, Australia and around the world I have discovered most people needed one of the following for each system. This is a guide only for you to investigate with your qualified naturopath or health professional.
Lots of good filtered water every day. (Eight glasses per day)
Boosting the Immune system. Echinacea, Astragalus Gold 3000, Young Living Immune power, or Australian Tea Tree Oil.
Vitamin C, Garlic, Colloidal Silver for natural antibiotic.
Vitamin B complex and Bio Zinc for stress. The body can use these up very quickly under stress and lack of them can cause lack of sex drive and prostate problems fellas.
Do not take vitamin B and C together as they will cancel each other out energetically.
Hydrochloric acid with pepsin tablet or organic acids for the stomach as this is important as there is very little acidity in the food in the USA.
I was told this by the vitamin/mineral doctor specialist. Probably why so much Coke is sold?
Gas, bad breath, constipation, etc can be caused by a lack of acid so you can safely take a tablet of hydrochloric acid and pepsin after a meal and if burns slightly you will probably not need it.
A glass of water will relieve the burning if this is the case. Talk to your health professional first as if you have been taking antacids they may have damaged the stomach lining and so this will not be an accurate test. **Do not take** with asprin, buzazolidin, inodicin, motrin or anti-inflammatories.
Frutin is a natural product from Denmark for relief of digestive disorders such as reflux and heartburn which creates a protective barrier between the stomach acid and sensitive tissues of the oesophagus and does not contain aluminium.
Absorbable calcium, Bio-magnesium, manganese and vitamin E are also high on the list and very important for the nerves and to stop osteoporosis in your spine.

Bio-magnesium on its own is good for muscular problems and painful cramps

Dehydroepiandrosterone (DHEA) may be one of the anti-aging hormones and have anti-cancer / anti-viral effects, prevent hardening of the arteries and heart attacks.

EDTA oral chelation works to lower your blood calcium to cut down on arterial build up of plaque that collects on the artery walls and literally chokes your system.

CO-Q 10 is having really good results for those with minor chest pains or heart problems, but not to be taken if on Wayfarin therapy without medical advice. It builds up / tones the heart muscles.

Shark cartilage 1000mg/Glucosamine sulfate 1000mg and Flax oil 1000mg (or Salmon oil 1000mg) and Lyprinol (Green Lipped Mussel Oil) is great when we are feeling stiff or for those arthritic pains. All these together with walking reasonably fast building up to 45 minutes every other day.

Wheat grass or Barley grass /green juice for chlorophyll and essential vitamins minerals etc.

If you have allergies to wheat products suggest you use the barley grass.

Royal Jelly will help balance the hormones, prevent premature ejaculation and regenerate the memory cells.

Gotu Kola and Brahmi is proving to be really good for clients with brain damage and for memory regeneration also.

St Johns Wort is having great results for depression although is not suitable mixing with some medications so be sure to ask your health professional before taking it.

Book St. Johns Wort Natures Blues Buster by Hyla Cass MD.

Eden GH1 and Super HGH all natural homeopathic oral sprays which simulate growth hormones for a natural booster for our pituitary gland to turn back the body's biological time clock 10-20 years in approximately six months according to the advertising. Reduce body fat and increase energy, better sleep, skin appearance, elasticity, and reverses aging, moods and depression.

Maca is a great hormone balancer for both male and females and is naturally grown at 14,000 feet elevation in unpolluted Peruvian Andes Mountains and is sold as an energy food sports food supplement. Good for mental clarity, increased energy, hormonal stabiliser and enhanced libido, rejuvenator. Not for ladies who have been diagnosed with cancer though!

Natures formula Colloidal minerals which are organic, plant derived and contains over 65 macro and trace minerals and is bio available. Readily digestible. (www.tjclark.com.au)

Natural progesterone instead of synthetic progestins or progestogens is doing a great job for the ladies during pre-menopause and menopause so find a Doctor who does the tests to see if you can apply it. Dr John R Lee MD book What Your Doctor May Not tell You About Menopause. Warner Books and Natural Progesterone: The multiple Roles of a Remarkable Hormone BLL Publishing, are two real eye openers. Menopause symptoms can affect you as young as 30, particularly if your body has been really stressed.

Iron from a vegetarian scource as this is non constipational, supports the haemoglobin, glucose energy levels, helps keep the blood at the right consistency, and stops anaemia.

Aloe Vera. If you grow a small plant and cut the plant leaf off whenever you get burnt and squeeze the white centre out and apply until it stops burning, it will do wonders for the skin and quite often there is no scarring.

An old 60-year-old friend of mine used to get at least 30-50 skin cancers cut off his face every year and since applying Aloe Vera once a day to his face he looks like a 40-year-old. He states he may look a little green at times but at least he does not suffer from the facial cancer anymore.

Ladies, if you have to use tampons then demand unbleached and all cotton, or risk from the bleaching process dioxin which is linked to potentially carcinogenic cancer.

The following is a guide only for you to have some idea of the uses of the vitamin and mineral substances. This is not a substitute for a good therapist who will be specializing in them but will give a good background for you to be able to ask intelligent questions about what you put in your body.

IMPORTANT SOURCES OF VITAMINS AND SYMPTOMS OF DEFICIENCY

Vitamin	Symptoms of Deficiency	Sources
A	night blindness, rough dry skin, ulcers, lack of resistance to infections, pain on urination, impaired vision, brittle nails and hair, stone formation, dandruff, various skin disorders	dandelion greens, carrots, apricots kale, sweet potato, pumpkin, parsley, mangoes, butter, broccoli, paw paw, eggs
B1 (Thiamine)	Irritability, instability, confusion, listlessness, loss of reflexes, muscular weakness, loss of appetite, constipation, intestinal troubles.	yeast, wheat germ, sunflower seeds, rice bran, pine nuts, peanuts, soybeans, cowpeas, brazil nuts, pecans, split peas, millet, buckwheat, oats, hazelnuts, lentils, rice, rye
B2 (Riboflavin)	Cracks and sores in corner of mouth, red sore tongue a feeling of grit inside eyelids, burning of eyes, sensitivity to light, scaling around nose, forehead and ears, vaginal itching, lack of stamina, oily skin.	Yeast, organ meats, almonds, wheat germ, mushrooms, millet, egg yolks, soy flour, split peas, sunflower seeds, fish, pine nuts, lentils, parsley, rice bran, cashews.

Vitamin	Symptoms of Deficiency	Sources
B3 (Niacin)	Depressed feeling, muscular weakness, general fatigue, loss of appetite indigestion, skin eruptions, tender gums, nervousness, tongue deep red, digestive problems	Yeast, rice bran, wheat bran, liver, fish, poultry, sesame seeds, sunflower seeds, brown rice, pine nuts, buck wheat, mushrooms, wheat germ, barley, almonds, split peas.
B5 (Pantothen)	Depression, weakness, easily stressed, intestinal acid, disturbances, numbness and tingling of hands and feet, dizziness.	Yeast, organ meats, split peas, mushrooms, soybean flour, eggs, oatmeal, buckwheat, sunflower seeds, lentils, cashews, broccoli, brown rice, and fish.
B 6 (Pyridoxine)	Fluid retention, loss of hair, cracks around mouth and eyes, sore lips and tongue, visual disturbances, nervousness irritability, slow learning	Yeast, sunflower seeds, wheat germ. soybeans, walnuts, fish, lentils, lima beans, buckwheat, brown rice, hazelnuts, bananas, avocados, egg yolk, rye, spinach.

Vitamin	Symptoms of Deficiency	Sources
B12	Anemia, soreness and weakness in arms and legs, decreased reflexes, sore tongue, numbness, stiffness, nervousness, tingling, apathy, loss of appetite, lack of concentration, hot and cold feelings, mental slowness.	Liver, kidney, milk, eggs, cheese, fish, wheat germ, soybeans, yeast alfalfa, comfrey, kelp.
P.Bio	(Works with C), varicose veins, bleeding gums, gums, bruise easily, fragile capillaries	Flavenoids, grapes, rose hips, citrus rinds, prunes, buckwheat, oranges, lemons blackcurrant, parsley, grapefruit, paw paw, tomato and broccoli
Fatty acids	Skin disorders, hair troubles, asthma, allergic	Unsaturated vegetable oils, wheat germ, seeds, nuts, fish, oils

Vitamin	Symptoms of Deficiency	Sources
K	Lowered vitality, nose bleeds, haemorrhages, miscarriages.	Turnip greens, broccoli, lettuce, cabbage, liver, spinach, alfalfa, sprouts, watercress, asparagus, cheese, butter oats, peas, beans, eggs
Biotin	Depression, extreme exhaustion, muscle pain, poor appetite, dry gray skin, disturbed nervous system	Egg yolk, beef liver, brewers yeast, soy flour, rice bran, walnuts, pecans, oats, lentils, sardines, almonds, brown rice, split peas, salmon
Choline	Liver degeneration, heart palpitations, ringing in ears, insomnia, dizziness, bleeding stomach ulcers.	Lecithin, egg yolk, liver, wheat germ, soy beans, brewers yeast, lentils, split peas, rice bran, oatmeal, brown rice, green peas, molasses

Vitamin	Symptoms of Deficiency	Sources
Inositol	Baldness, constipation, high cholesterol, eczema, eye problems	Lecithin, wheat germ, navy beans, rice bran, whole wheat, citrus, brewers yeast, molasses, soy beans, peas, split peas, lentils, brown rice
C Ascorbic Acid	Easy bleeding and bruising, anemia, colds, infections, shortness of breath, gout, slow ACID healing, lack of resistance	Red chilli peppers, guavas, capsicum, kale, parsley, broccoli, brussel sprouts, mustard greens, watercress, cauliflower, rose hip, tomatoes, citrus, strawberries, paw paw
D Choleacal iferol	Bone deformity, teeth and gum problems, lack of resilience in skin and tissues, rickets, insomnia	Fish liver oil, organ meats, egg yolk, salmon, tuna, herring, butter, sprouted seeds(if exposed to sunlight)sunflower seeds, mushrooms, natural cheeses, sunlight action on skin

Vitamin	Symptoms of Deficiency	Sources
E	Enlarged prostate, sterility, kidney disease, dull dry hair, fat deposits in muscles, varicose veins, general weakness	Wheat germ oil, sunflower seeds, vegetable oils, seeds, nuts, wheat germ, butter, brown rice, whole grain

IMPORTANT SOURCES OF MINERALS AND SYMPTOMS OF DEFICIENCY

Mineral	Function	Symptoms of Deficiency	Sources
Alumin-ium		**Excess is damaging** if it accumulates slowly over many years. **Excess** symptoms: Intestinal disturbances, senile dementia, headaches, hyperactivity, dermatitis and inflammation of sweat glands.	Aluminum cooking utensils, aluminum foil, tobacco smoke, antacids, antiperspirants, aspirin compounds, baking powder.
Calcium	Needed for bones, cartilages, proper blood clotting, nerve and muscle functioning and activates, necessary for acid base balance	Nervousness and irritability, osteoporosis, excess menstruation, stunted growth, leg cramps, soft bones, heart palpitations.	Kelp, cheese, carob, almonds, yogurt, parsley, tofu, figs, sunflower seeds, buckwheat, sesame seeds

Mineral	Function	Symptoms of Deficiency	Sources
Chromium	Stimulates enzymes involved with glucose metabolism, increases effectiveness of insulin.	Glucose intolerance (disturbance in sugar metabolism.)	Yeast, whole wheat, potatoes, wheat germ, green pepper, apples, butter
Fluoride		Tooth decay, spinal curvature, weakened bones, prolapse.	Carrots, dandelion, spinach, seafood.
Iodine	Aids in development and function of thyroid gland, plays important role in regulating the body.	Sluggishness, irritability	Kelp, seafood, garlic, onions, eggs, pineapple, spinach.

Mineral	Function	Symptoms of Deficiency	Sources
Iron	Its major function is to combine with protein and copper to make hemoglobin, the coloring matter of red blood cells. Iron also help indirectly to transport oxygen throughout the body.	Deficiency symptoms: Anemia, pale skin, fatigue, brittle nails and breathing problems.	Kelp, yeast molasses, pumpkin seeds, wheat germ, sunflower seeds, millet, parsley, cashews, almonds, brazil nuts, pecans, leafy green vegetables, lentils, tofu, brown rice.
Magne-sium	Aids in bone growth and is necessary for proper functioning of nerves and muscles.	Deficiency symptoms: Muscle cramps, nerve irritability, convulsions, digestive troubles, irregular heartbeat.	Kelp, wheat germ, almonds, cashews, molasses, yeast, buckwheat, brazil nuts, peanuts, millet, pecan nuts, rye, tofu, spinach, beet greens, brown rice, figs, dates, parsley, sunflower seeds.

Mineral	Function	Symptoms of Deficiency	Sources
Manga- nese	Necessary for bone develop- ment, normal pancreas functioning, important for brain func- tioning, aids in metabolism of fats and carbohydrates.	Bone malforma- tion, dizziness, impaired growth, depressed sexual function.	Pecans, brazil nuts, almonds, barley, rye, buck- wheat, wheat, walnuts, Oats, peanuts, raisins, millet, brown rice
Phos- phorus			Yeast, wheat bran, pumpkin seeds, soybeans, rye, almonds, cashews, mil- let, pecans, kelp, brown rice, eggs, cottage cheese, lentils, raisins
Silicon	Essential for healthy hair, skin and nails.	Suppurations, brittle hair and nails	Oat straw tea, parsnip, spin- ach, cucumber, strawberries, sunflower seeds, onion, aspara- gus, brown rice.

Mineral	Function	Symptoms of Deficiency	Sources
Sodium	Aids digestion and helps keep other minerals soluble. Helps remove carbon dioxide from the body. Involved in muscular contractions.	Dehydration, salt hunger.	Meat, fish, legumes, kelp, olives, salt, celery, spinach, onion, garlic, sesame seeds, carrot, parsley, sunflower seeds, cabbage, eggs.
Zinc	Necessary for healing wound and during infection and stress. Needed for insulin productions	Deficiencies: Hair loss, diarrhea, restricted growth and sexual development, nail changes, decreases immune strength, weakness.	Oysters, pumpkin seeds, pecans, brazil nuts, egg yolk, hazelnuts, fish

John Chamberlin

Mineral	Function	Symptoms of Deficiency	Sources
Potas-sium	Necessary for nerve stimulation and healthy skin and adrenal gland health. Stimulates kidneys in waste elimination.	Fluid retention, muscular weakness, nervousness.	Kelp, sunflower seeds, wheat germ, almonds, raisins, parsley, brazil nuts, dates, avocados, pecans, soybeans, spinach, millet, potato, broccoli, banana, meats, squash, carrots, lentils, paw paw, oranges

Hair Chemicals

Hair dyes do a wonderful job but please check the labels as the wrong BREW can cause massive depression and headaches. No use looking great with too much depression and tiredness to get out and enjoy being beautiful is there? There are some really great hair dyes on the natural counter now days. They are not as greasy and oily, or in the horrid colors they used to be. The colors have changed with the times. Ask a female naturopath what she uses and the same time ask her what brand of shampoo she uses too.

If you will not change for any reason, help your hair a little. One of the best things for your hair is apple cider vinegar. Pour an eighth of a glass (about ¼ inch), fill the glass up to the top with warm water and after washing out all the shampoo and conditioner, rinse the whole glass of cider vinegar mix through your hair and towel dry lightly. Let it dry in your hair. The slight odour will shortly disappear. Cider vinegar is not offensive and will keep you hair really silky and free from dandruff. A good tip from a natural beauty therapist.

Acrylic Nails

In our plan for beauty these fashion option **stick ons** may cause some serious health problems.

Many ladies are experiencing allergic reactions to the chemicals from the artificial nails, and others are developing infections between the artificial nail and the finger. In some cases it has been mild skin and nail irritation while others have reported their entire natural nail falling off. At least five to 10 per cent have problems such as chemical reaction, abnormal shaped regrowth as the matrix of the nail has been affected. Infection, fungal, yeast, bacteria infections for those who have their hands in water.

How could you wash yourself properly without getting your hands in water?

If you must wear them! Good news! There are some 100 per cent organic nails now being made so check it out. They are made by mixing a liquid monomer with a powder polymer and then this moulding of acrylic compound is put onto the natural nail. They look good however natural is still best.

Parasites

Investigate buying a Zapper which will kill, or at least render harmless or less active, parasites in your system. This little black box is not approved for use on humans as it would cost too much to get approval under the rules and regulations from the FDA and the AMA.

My experience has shown really phenomenal results. Others I know who own one have achieved similar results. Most people do not want to talk about this subject but if you are in a state of dis- ease then you not only need to purchase one but also take the herbal dose of Black Walnut Hull tincture, Cloves and Wormwood from your local Naturopath.

Orders for Rascal or similar herbs from Kroeger Herb Products Co., Inc. of 1122 Pearl St. Boulder, Colorado 80302. Phone # 303-443-0261. Information for these can be obtained or purchased from most leading health food stores or naturopaths.

If you can't get a copy write to Alternative Therapies at PO Box 11627 Honolulu Hawaii or phone # 808-942-7128, or Self Health Resource Center at 757 Emory St. # 508 Imperial Beach CA 91932 USA, PH 619-429-4408

The book with the information about this incredible little machine is called A Cure for all Diseases by Hulda Clark. Hulda found during experimentation that in just about all diseases she found parasites present and incredible results occurred to better the health of clients when the parasites were eradicated. She found that parasites could not stand a certain type of electronic wave and would die rather quickly. The book explains how to make one yourself if you are so inclined. The herbs are to kill those so deeply buried in your system that the shock does not penetrate like eyes and testicles. I have heard and seen first hand how many little miracles have happened to improve health resulting from using this machine. One guy I knew used to cough all the time and after years of nervous coughing tried a Zapper for another symptom in his stomach. Imagine his surprise when three days later he coughed up an inch long worm and has not coughed since. You girls are not off the hook as a client of mine had complained of soreness in the pubic area. Gynaecological inspections had produced no help so she borrowed a machine. Without going into detail she had a little surprise the next morning and hasn't had the same problem again. She has since bought her own machine to use in three to six monthly follow-ups.

Colloidal Silver Machines

Purchase some colloidal silver from your local health food store or naturopath and take it according to the instructions. Colloidal silver was used near the beginning of the 1900s as an antibiotic until making it became too expensive. It was sold at approximately $40 an ounce so other antibiotics were developed and used. According to my reading and experience about colloidal silver it seems to stop the mutation of most diseases, toxins and viruses with no apparent side effects except some constipation which to my mind is the body keeping the toxins together to put out of the body.

With all the threat of being exposed to weird and wonderful diseases from terrorists, unenlightened people and misguided countries, I for one will always have one of these machines to give me a fighting chance to have the health I was born with and deserve.

These little machines consist of two silver electrodes and a power supply and when attached to the power scource the two 99.9 per cent silver electrodes are put into water. While one electrode gives off little air bubbles, a tiny cloud of colloidal silver comes off the other one. It only takes 20 - 25 minutes, depending on how much colloidal silver you make with your own machine, which to me is preferential to paying ridiculous prices.

I suggest you purchase a bottle of high quality colloidal silver, check the silver against your system and if this is what your body wants and needs then purchase your own manufacturing machine and make your own colloidal silver. Take as according to the instructions. Remember that sometimes a healing crisis takes place for the first few days as the toxins can hit the bloodstream to be put out of the body as quickly as possible. Call your health provider or counsellor before persevering with this.
Follow the instructions please! DO NOT OVERDOSE!

These colloidal silver machines can be purchased from the writer or from LIVING FROM VISION at PO Box 1530 Stanwood WA 98292 USA. PH 360-387-9846 or Alternative Therapies Research phone 808-942-7128. They can be purchased for approximately $100 to$145 depending on the instrument. There are some cheaper machines so please satisfy yourself about the integrity of the instrument before purchasing.
The Food and Drug Administration has stated that because colloidal silver is a pre 1938 drug by 50 years and it may be marketed as the FDA has no jurisdiction regarding a pure mineral element. This decision may have changed since this book was written so check this out with the supplier.

Prior to 1938 colloidal silver was administered in just about every way that modern drugs are administered. It was injected, intravenously and intramuscularly, used as a gargle for throat conditions, as a douche, taken orally and applied topically on sensitive tissues and dropped in the eyes.

Science Digest article, March 1978 entitled Our Mightiest Germ Fighter by Jim Powell reported: Thanks to eye opening research, silver is emerging as a wonder of modern medicine. An antibiotic kills perhaps half-a-dozen kinds of disease organisms, but silver kills some 650 resistant strains that fail to develop. Moreover, silver is virtually non- toxic.

Dr Harry Margraf of St. Louis a pioneering silver researcher states, Silver is the best all round germ fighter we have.

There are hundreds of good things said about colloidal silver but its best if you research it yourself to see what I mean.

The following are some of the benefits, conditions and pathogens that colloidal silver was documented and used before 1938.

Acne
Arthritis
Athletes Foot
Bladder Inflammation
Burns
B. Tuberculosis
B. Hepatitis
C. Colitis
Cystitis
Diphtheria
Dermatitis
Diabetes
Dysentery
Ear infections
Eustachian Tubes
Eczema
Fibrosis
Furunculosis
Gonorrheal Herpes
Gonorrhea
Impetigo
Influenza
Intestinal trouble
Keratitis
Leprosy
Lupus
Lymphangitis
Malaria
Meniere's Symptoms
Meningitis
Nemasthenia
Ophthalmology
Canine Parvo Virus
Pneumonia
Pleurisy

Prostate
Rheumatism
Ringworm
Rhinitis
Scarlatina
Schorrhea
Septic Ulcers
Sepsis
Septicemia
Skin Cancer
Shingles
Soft Sores
Spruce
Staph Infections
Strep Infections
Subdues Inflammation
Tuberculosis
Tonsillitis
Toxemia
Typhoid
Trench foot
Ulcers
Warts
Whooping Cough
Yeast Infections

The following was copied from a commercial brand flyer from Silver Wings Colloidal Silver to show the small doses that are necessary. This brand was considered to be very pure by those recommending it and gave good results.

SILVER WINGS COLLOIDAL SILVER
Natural Antibiotic - Anti-viral - Anti-fungal

Adult Usage   Always dilute with pure distilled, de-ionized or reverse osmosis water.

Children   0-6 years ¼ adult amount
7-12 years ½ adult amount

Acute Infection   2 teaspoons per day for 7 days, then 1 teaspoon per day. If symptoms persist, consult your health care professional.

Chronic Infection   2 teaspoons for 10 days, then 1 teaspoon per day for 3 to 6 months, as directed by your health care professional.

Tooth and Gum Infection 1 teaspoon in 3 ounces of water and rinse vigorously, then swallow liquid. Do this once daily until gums are healthy. Add ½ teaspoon to liquid in water pick type units and clean as usual if desired.

Eyes   For short-term usage, put one drop silver to three parts water in the eyes each night.

Ears   A few drops in the ear, however, the ENT Colloidal Silver Formula is more effective for this usage.

Sore Throat   1 teaspoon in 3 ounces of water, gargle morning and night. Swallow liquid. Use until symptom free.

Vaginal Infection   2 teaspoons in 8 ounces of water. Douche daily for seven days.

Herpes Inflammation Use full strength topically on herpes blisters hourly until gone. Use internally as for acute infections.

Topical Use Apply directly to cuts, scrapes, warts, ashes, acne, mosquito bites and many other skin problems.

Water Purification 1 teaspoon per gallon and shake well.

Digestive Aid Drink one 8-oz. glass of the above mixture over a days time, especially with meals. This will eliminate fermentation.

Preventative and Maintenance Usage Silver Wings Colloidal Silver may be diluted 50 times with pure water to reduce to the same potency as most colloidal silvers on the market.

For Animals: Depending on the size of the ear canal, use a dropper to put colloidal silver down the throat, or just put it in your pets food or water.

For Plants: For bacterial, fungal and viral attacks on plants, simply spray diluted silver on the leaves. Mix one tablespoon per quart of water.

Disclaimer: Neither manufacturer or seller makes any claims as to any specific benefits occurring from the use of colloidal silver. Information conveyed herein is based on records and research for your information only and is not meant to imply that you will experience similar benefits or results. Any benefits or results derived from the use of colloidal silver are subjective due to variable individual health factors and metabolic differences that tend to make the formula more or less adaptogenic. Some individuals may experience a cleansing reaction characterized by tiredness, digestive disturbances or other symptoms. If at any time severe discomfort is experienced or symptoms persist, discontinue use and consult your health care professional.

Natural Health Research Group
1-800-242-0828 USA

Allergies

Check whether you have allergies to feathers and if so get rid of your feather pillows and feather bed coverall. Don't want to get rid of it? Then move into another room for a few weeks that has hypo allergenic pillows and freshly washed blankets and bed linen to see if you can breathe easier. It may not be the feathers but some chemical in the pillows to stop the bugs eating them and to get rid of lice. Birds do get lice you know.

While you are at it, if you have birds as pets, move them into another room or into the garage for a few days to see if your allergies are better. Also clean up the place the pet normally habitats. If the pet is still affecting you then find a good home for it and get a different kind of pet. It is amazing the number of people who have asthma and feather allergies who have birds, or fur allergies from cats and dogs and a house full of cats and dogs living with them. Change your pet. They won't want to see you miserable either because of them.

A lady in Phoenix was being eaten alive. Her whole body was covered with bites from no see ums, which are like a midge or sandfly, and she still allowed her dogs to go out and play near the irrigation canals and then sleep on her bed at night. Quality of life for whom? I love animals but there needs to be common sense or make a decision to be miserable and stop looking for a cure.

A kinesiologist can help disconnect and help balance hay fever and most allergies as I thankfully have found out for myself.
Allergies are a whole science in itself so suggest instead of reinventing the wheel suggest you purchase The Allergy Bible by Linda Gamlin (www.allergy-intolerance.com)

Asthma/Ionisers/Air Cleaners

If you still get asthma, or find it hard to breathe, get your favorite chiropractor to check your back as it may be out of alignment somewhere around the first, second and third thoracic vertebrae. Purchase an Al-an-ra therapeutic ioniser or similar to energise the room and kill all the bacteria, dust mites etc. in the room especially where you sleep. This can be purchased from Bionic Products Pty Ltd 63 Manly Drive Robina Qld. 4226 Australia. Ph 07-5593-1122.

If you can't get one of these, most drug stores have negative ionisers for sale at approximately $100 to $120 each that will do a whole room. You might well ask what this does.

Have you ever been out in the country after rain or beside a waterfall and smelt that fresh clean smell and noticed that breathing seems easier as there is no dust in the air. That is what an ioniser does. You will be amazed at the dust, pollens and garbage in the air that drop on the floor or in the filters so you don't have to breathe it in. I had one in my hotel room whenever I stayed longer than one night and the rubbish collected in the filters at times was amazing. When travelling on an aircraft I have a small air purifier around my neck to avoid bacteria contamination from other sometimes inconsiderate sick coughing people. I highly recommend this as it has worked for me. With all the viruses that are in the confined space of an aircraft today, the number of people travelling and the number of new viruses being found, aircraft filter systems cannot stop the spread of viral strains. Recent outbreaks of deadly, highly contagious viruses such as Ebola and Haemorrhagic fever have occurred that are untreatable. These ancient pathogens could mutate to airborne forms such as occurred in a well documented outbreak just outside Washington DC. Reportedly, airborne Hauntovirus traced to the Han River in Korea had broken out in New Mexico and California. Should any of these viruses be carried aboard an international airline, travelling without adequate personal protection in filtering systems could be very dangerous. These life forms have been mutating for millions of years and even though they are microscopic they have the capacity to decimate a human being.

The Center for Disease control in The United States has confirmed four cases of tuberculosis infection from air travel. I believe it is only a matter of time before a major outbreak of some mysterious disease will come from some remote country. I am prepared using the Air Supply Unit and I might add, this little air purifier has stopped me getting some really heavy illnesses while travelling next to another passenger with a full-blown flu or virus. On previous experience I would have ended up with the virus within days.

This air purifier called AIR SUPPLY can be bought from Wein Products Inc., 115 W. 25 th St., Los Angeles CA. 9007 USA Ph 213-749-6049, which also provided most of the following information about the environment.

If breathing problems still persist then go to a counselor or hypnotherapist to find out the emotional problem behind the lack of life (breath) in your life.

John Chamberlin

SOME POISONS IN THE HOME OR OFFICE WHICH CAN CAUSE BREATH PROBLEMS, DEPRESSION, TIREDNESS.

Chemical	Found In	Causes
Benzene	Paint, new carpets, new drapes, upholstery	Headaches, eye and skin irritation and cancer
Ammonia	Tobacco smoke, cleaning supplies	Eye and skin irritation, headaches, nose bleeds, sinus problems
Chloroform	New drapes, upholstery, new carpeting	Headaches, asthma attacks, dizziness, eye irritation, skin irritation
Formaldehyde	Tobacco smoke, plywood cabinets, furniture, particleboard, office dividers, new carpets and drapes, wallpaper and paneling.	Eye and skin irritation, drowsiness, fatigue, respiratory problems, memory loss, depression, gynecological problems, cancer
Benzopyrene	Tobacco smoke	Asthma attacks, eye and skin irritation, sinus problems and lung cancer
Hydrocarbons	Tobacco smoke, gas burners, furnaces	Headaches, fatigue, nausea, dizziness, breathing difficulty
Trichlorethylene	Paints, glue, furniture, wallpaper	Headaches, eye and skin irritation, Respiratory irritation
Xylene	Paint, new carpets, cleaning supplies	Headaches, dizziness, fatigue

This does not mean that you should do something drastic, it helps you realize if you are sensitive enough to question your surroundings before blaming yourself for being diseased and where possible make changes. Perhaps you can now see the importance of an ioniser.

One of the age-old remedies for blocked nose and sinuses is to get some sea salt (natural salt water is preferred) and sterilize it by boiling in a little water, pour to a small glass bottle and add a pinch of Epsom salts. Lay your head back while standing near a basin, hold one nostril closed with one finger and using a sterilized eyedropper, sniff the sterilised salt water up the other nostril. It may make you cough, as the salt-water hits the back of your throat but you will benefit by losing the gunk that comes free. You will need to repeat this at least three times each side. If the solution burns dilute the water a little next time or follow with pure water. Yes, it does hurt a little but has the same effect as going for a swim in the ocean. If you can remember going swimming you will also remember your runny nose as the salt water did its work up your nose when your head went under the waves. This works far better than all the other nose sprays, is natural and is not habit forming.

Tea Tree Oil

Skin rashes, athletes' foot and fungus (smelly feet) respond really well to the Australian Tea Tree Essential Oil known as melaleuca. A really good book Australian Tea Tree Oil First Aid Handbook by Cynthia Olsen was published which describes melaleuca as a cure all for most things.

Tea Tree Oil was taken internally by Naturopath Karen Cutter to show the oil is safe. She took up to 120 drops a day for up to three months and uses it successfully for the treatment of candida etc. as it had the effects of being an antiseptic and could slow the bad or unbalanced yeast growth. The taste though would have been horrendous.

According to my sources the so-called authorities have recently required a poison label on the bottle with no change to the ingredients. This stuff must be really good! I use a teaspoon of Aromatherapy oil with about 10 drops of melaleuca high grade in the bath for my skin and also put a few drops of melaleuca in hair shampoo for skin care and to restrict dandruff on the scalp. It has been used very successfully on women with trichomonal vaginitis, thrush, cervicitis and insect bites. Ask your own naturopath or homeopathic doctor and make your own inquiries as to the potency of your bottle of Melaleuca before trying this. Use it a little at a time to see that you are satisfied with the difference it makes and to ensure you have no reactions. For those of us with a fungus under our nails, especially feet, where the nail bed is affected, great results have come from cleaning out as far as you can under the nail without destroying the nail bed. Then drop a drop of melaleuca under the nail night and morning until better. There is a great write-up in the medical Journal of Australia January 1930 p417 called A New Australian Germicide by E. Humphrey. Calamine lotion is also very good for most heat rashes.

Sauna/Spa/Massage for Our Skin and Muscles.

Our skin is our largest organ and know that we are meant to perspire or sweat. I was always told horses sweat. The reason for perspiring is not only to cool the body's blood temperature but also to help eliminate toxins from the body that cannot come through other excretory channels. One of the most pleasant ways to enjoy this is to go with a friend to a sauna and spa bathhouse. Sit in the steam, getting hotter and hotter by the minute, until you can't take the heat any more then go out and have a cool shower, or if it's snowing outside jump in the snow and cool off. (Sounds romantic, but it's not, as it can freeze the b--- off a brass monkey. Then go back and repeat it all over again two or three times, **providing you have had a heart check beforehand** by your local general practitioner and have a clearance form from him or her.
Do not do this if you have a heart condition without the advice of your doctor. The sauna is really good for stimulating your immune and muscular system, and even though you may be very tired after,

you will usually awake next morning feeling really refreshed whether your partner stayed or not. By the way, I believe that lovemaking is like the fountain of youth and is fantastic for energizing the immune system. The benefits of lovemaking are well known by doctors and therapists alike who prescribe for chronic immune problem sufferers and recommend they make love a lot more as it stimulates the system back to better health. Touch is very important to everyone for health and well-being and if you don't like to be touched, you may not want to hear this, but know you have a problem and need to see a therapist about it. Get a therapeutic massage.

A spa is a bath that has air jets into the water space at various outlets directed towards your body that make the water very turbulent. You would normally be lying in warm water with your head out of the water unless you like snorkelling. The weight of water being pushed around stimulates the muscle tissue, making your body move. The body perspires and this can be really pleasant and stimulating with or in company of someone special. Especially with a cool drink close at hand in an unbreakable cup. Who said getting healthy couldn't be fun?

The Australian made Vibrosaun is an economic machine you can lie down in and listen to music with your head out of the heat and still simulate exercise without putting stress on the body.
It heats the body like a sauna and a vibrating board under you makes the body move and be stimulated to perspire, improve muscle tone, help eliminate body wastes, relieve tension and stress, back pains, etc. Great for those who need to lose weight and are not very mobile or recovering from an operation.

A therapeutic massage with aromatherapy oils by a certified aroma therapist/massage therapist after a spa will leave you as though in an altered state.

The Poor man's sauna really works!
Don't do this unless your heart is in good condition, as the process will make it work and get it pumping hard. As some of these sauna

and spa rooms can be rather expensive. I suggest you find trusted friends who is not offended by nudity and ask them to stay with you and help you.

I say trusted friends as you need to know that they are not going through your stuff when you are resting and out to it on the floor. They need to be there if you need a hand as you can feel rather weak on coming out of the blankets, besides you will **relax** much better if you can trust them. Lay two to three blankets flat on the floor, then wet a sheet in cold water and lay it flat on top of the blankets. Undress to your birthday suit, and lay straight with your arms by your sides on the cold sheet with a small pillow for your head. Have your friends then wrap you tightly in the sheet first, and then with the blankets until you are in a cocoon like state. You may shiver a little until you body warms the sheet and blankets. Stay in this for approximately 20-25 minutes then have your friends wake you up and help you out, as you may be rather weak. Then give you a cup of warm tea and wrap you up in something warm, before you have a warm shower and relax. It is necessary for your friends not let you go over 30 minutes. Be prepared for a horrible stench as your body will have osmosis effect and drop into the blankets a lot of toxins through the perspiration. Yes, you may even perspire after the body warms up in the blankets.

Massage

I hear bad things all the time about massage therapy from uninformed, unenlightened people. Admittedly there are in my opinion a whole bunch of misinformed people who cannot trust their own emotions, don't trust themselves and are not comfortable with their own sexuality and have to condemn anything they personally cannot comprehend or understand. There are also misguided over sexed people (bad self image again, or lacking security) who give massage a terrible name and from what I have heard at most of these clubs, give a really lousy massage and they are only interested in one thing. Did I hear greed or money mentioned? However the lights are on and getting brighter and I can tell you from experience over the last 20 years that using Swedish therapeutic and deep tissue massage as one of my natural tools to get people healthy is one of the best modes used to get the body well. Massage is one of the best!

Therapeutic massage is **not** sexual massage! You are draped and covered at all times so your modesty is kept intact. A professional massage therapist's goal is to have all your body, mind and emotions really relaxed when he has finished, so why would he annoy you and get you hyped up, if nudity is an issue to you. If this does happen, and you are not comfortable, talk about it, and if it cannot be resolved, get dressed, walk out of there and find a better same sex therapist. Sometimes, however, a massage may be painful as the certified therapist works and kneads the muscle tissue to get all the stale blood or toxins out of the muscle tissue to get the immune system back into the best order/health that can be obtained in the session. Inside our bodies we have what is called lymphatic fluid which is a clear watery like substance that diffuses through the veins taking food /oxygen to the cells of the body and bringing waste back to the excretory organs. For good health, these ducts rely on muscle flexing to motivate the fluid along the collapsible channels, and massage, exercise plus a fast heartbeat is imperative to help this process.
If this doesn't happen, a build up of tension and blood toxins accumulate and push on the nerves in the body causing phantom pains in some areas of the body. See diagram on Chiropractic chart. Massage will help the lymphatic system recover as it gets the blood to flow again bringing back flexibility.

A really noticeable lymphatic imbalance is little lumps in or under the side of the breast, the armpits, on the inside of the thigh above the groin area, or on the side of the neck. Dowager's hump on the shoulders behind the neck usually on overweight people is a lymphatic problem. This can be corrected with first manipulating correcting the shoulders and ligaments back to their natural positioning and realigning the first and second thoracic vertebrae into place and lots of massage on the afflicted area to send the fluid on its merry way. Sometimes it is genetic also.

While I am on this subject, ladies, it is imperative to massage your breasts every day while in the shower as there can be considerable build up in the lymphatics when you carry a heavy bag over the shoulder and stop the natural flow. I have stopped many operations of breast cancer by opening up the drainage areas around the rib cage and under the breast tissue where possible and the lumps most times dissipate and seldom return. Remember that a medical person who is diagnosing makes money doing an operation and can get sued if he says it is not cancer, if it grows again later. It is called covering your ass.

There is a lot of controversy on the validity of mammography now and it appears that even the National Cancer Institute was reported in the New York Times as willing to say that mammograms don't work. Save yourself the hurt, the embarrassment, the expense and the danger and replace it with regular self-breast exams or have a scan done by digital infrared thermal imaging if you are worried. know more about this at www.ThermoscanAustralia.com.au.

Tight bras constricting breast tissue, hampers lymph drainage and causes degeneration and if you need to wear one then try to pick one without a steel under wire which can change the molecular structure that causes damming of the lymph fluid. Do not wear a bra to bed. Book: Bra and Breast Cancer by Soma and Syd Singer.

Dr Gofman a nuclear physicist and a medical doctor, is being reported as saying mammograms / X - rays cause cancer. His book Radiation from medical procedures in the Pathogenesis of Cancer and Ischemic heart disease strongly indicates that over 50 per cent of Cancer today and over 60 per cent of the death rate from Ischemic heart disease today are X-Ray induced.

By the way, if you have a job that you are sitting down a lot and your thighs are getting larger round the pocket area, massage can help reduce this. Women will notice men do not get this much unless really overweight. Your body is much softer because of the female hormones and so by sitting in the one position all the time, the tissues under your legs get squashed. The blood goes round the side of the edge of the chair and builds up in tissue and fat cells there on the thighs. Get a chair that takes the pressure off the legs and you can adjust up and down. Organise yourself to walk round for at least five minutes every hour and have a massage weekly until your shape is back. It may help relieve the carpel tunnel syndrome too by moving the height of your chair up and down.

A massage will normally take at least 1- 1½ hours. If I have one or two good massages a week my body, mind and emotions are at a perfect optimum and my body is very flexible. Massage is one of the oldest and simplest of all therapies and has been used for thousands of years. It is still one of the best and most beneficial ways of keeping the body free of stress and toxicity and a very efficient way of relieving pain, stiffness and repairing injuries. It can relax the body, and realign the skeletal system, muscular system, cardiovascular, respiratory, digestive, endocrine, lymphatic and nervous systems, as well as relieving congestion and restoring balance to the body, mind and emotions if done right. During the course of my training and working for 20 years in the field of healing I have noticed that the people who looked the fittest in their older years were the ones who had a massage at least once a week, almost like a religion and going to church. If you think that you cannot afford the $40-50 a week, then make inquiries to find out who teaches a good therapeutic massage, get a friend interested to learn with you so you can have massage when you practice.

Personally I would rather fast one day a week to have the money for my massage. There are many forms of massage being taught now like Swedish Therapeutic, Reflexology, Metamorphic, Aromatherapy, Rolfing, Polarity therapy, Shiatsu, Ka Huna, Chinese, etc. They are all good but I find the quickest result for me has been the deep tissue Swedish massage while occasionally for chronic back pain, sciatica using a natural anti-inflammatory pain cream and a Medic 2000 tens machine to loosen up stubborn muscles and ligaments.

This combined with the physio-movement therapies that involve natural stretching to put everything back into alignment. Regressional work, emotional release work and electronic acupuncture are also very good to loosen up a back problem. Many doctors now suggest

that after a major operation massage it is important to the healing process to regenerate the muscle tissue and help relieve the stiffness. Most major healing centers now give their clients a massage a day.
A massage a day keeps the doctor away.

Medihoney

For those cuts abrasions and minor wounds this antibacterial honey forms a protective barrier over the wound helping to create a moist healing environment and is sterile not like commercial honeys. It acts to lift debris from the wound and stops the dressing from sticking to the wound, minimising pain and damage to the wound. (www.medihoney.com)

Aromatherapy
- great for massage, or room airo-matics.

Aromatherapy is the use of pure essential oils distilled from herbs, flowers, roots, woods and resins that are usually kept in dark bottles for preservation and to avoid adverse effects of light. Their properties assist the body's natural healing processes. To list all the therapeutic properties is almost impossible in a manual and the properties listed here are intended as a general guide to effective self help and healing.
Serious problems should of course be referred to the appropriate practitioners.

For further information on the subject refer to AROMATHERAPY - The Use of Plant Essences in Healing by Raymond Lautie D. Sc. and Andre Passebec M.D. D.Ps which is a very helpful reference for correct dosage etc.

CONCENTRATED PURE ESSENTIAL OILS

BERGAMOT is obtained from the rind of the fruit. It is used in many perfume preparations and makes pleasant bath oil. It is helpful in cases of bronchitis as it clears the bronchial tubes and is a useful remedy for minimizing or prevention of cold sores (herpes virus) if applied direct to the lips as soon as the symptoms present themselves. Also an antiseptic for the urinary tract, a deodorant, an antidepressant and a leucorrhoea remedy.

BLACK PEPPER popular with the men. Stimulating particularly on the digestive tract and claimed to be an aphrodisiac. A tonic for the spleen and aids muscle tone and also relieves flatulence.

CALENDULA (Marigold) for external application for cuts, boils, sores or other open wounds.

CHAMOMILE an anti-inflammatory and anti-allergic agent. A gout and rheumatic remedy when used with camphor. For teething problems gently rub the child's cheeks. Vertigo remedy. A pleasant bath oil when combined with geranium and lavender.
Useful for muscular aches after sporting activities.

CAMPHOR obtained from the wood. A first aid remedy to always keep in the house especially with children around. Immediate application to injuries such as bangs and sprains helps to prevent swelling and bruising. Alleviates pain.
A strong stimulant which **must not be used during pregnancy.**

CEDARWOOD obtained from the wood, and together with juniper is a wonderful natural remedy for cystitis and related kidney/ bladder problems - see Juniper. Can be taken internally at the first signs, 2 drops three times a day as well as drinking plenty of fluids. Useful for oily skin and for acne in facial rinsing acts as an antiseptic and will relieve itching. Helpful in the relief of rheumatism because of its diuretic action.

CLARY SAGE This is a popular oil and has a lovely aromatic perfume. Obtained from the herb, it is a very powerful relaxant and should not be used prior to driving a vehicle as it induces drowsiness. It is a sore throat remedy, a uterine tonic and for vertigo 3 drops on brown sugar sucked slowly 3 times a day.

A small amount massaged into the cheeks at night helps insomnia sufferers.

CYPRESS distilled from the cones. A powerful antispasmodic, useful for painful periods and for excessive discharge of body fluids. e.g. excessive menstrual flow and incontinence.
A tonic for the veins and used as a varicose vein remedy in a massage oil if applied very gently.
During flu epidemics use on a handkerchief or in a room spray.

EUCALYPTUS An anti-viral agent. As an insect repellent and protection against bites and stings use 1-2 drops on the hands or wrists. Use for all types of fever, a chest and sinus rub when used in massage oil (not near the eyes) and a remedy for cold sore and blister type skin eruptions. Ideal for inhalations, arthritis and rheumatism.

FENNEL (Sweet) Antispasmodic and remedy for hiccough, constipation, obesity and menopausal problems. A natural cough mixture - see First Aid section. Anti-wrinkle properties. A few drops taken will disguise the taste and odour of garlic.
Also used for aniseed flavouring in food.

FRANKINCENSE A good inhalant and lung tonic which deepens the breathing. Useful for catarrh conditions in the body. Helpful for piles when combined with juniper in the bath.
Very popular as a perfume.

GERANIUM A pleasant perfume. Used for all skin types including dry eczema and burns (for weeping eczema see Juniper) and a well-known treatment of ulcerated wounds, menopausal problems and gastric ulcers.

GINGER obtained from the root. A very warming oil useful for backaches in a massage oil. Promotes perspiration and is helpful at the onset of a cold.
For flatulence take 4 drops on a little brown sugar after each meal.

HYSSOP a blood pressure regulator, not to be used by epileptic sufferers. An expectorant and reliever of bronchial spasm. Alleviates hypertension, it's a nerve tonic. Helps to reduce scar tissue, an ingredient of chartreuse and expensive perfumes. For sore throats take 3 drops on brown sugar 3 times a day.

JUNIPER obtained from the berries has antirheumatic and diuretic properties.
As with cedarwood this is an excellent remedy for cystitis and related problems. Cedarwood and juniper combined give even better results and used in conjunction with the Juniper/Cedarwood/Bergamot massage oil will give effective relief. A remedy for gout and colic and useful for oily skin and, toning the skin and stimulating the circulation. Helps to keep bronchial tubes clear. For weeping eczema bathe in a solution of 2 per cent juniper in boiled water. Juniper can be taken internally in small amounts.

LAVENDER A must for every first aid cabinet. Obtained from the flowers, can be used for all skin types. Wonderful remedy for burns, inflammations, cuts, grazes etc. acting as a rejuvenating agent to the skin. Effective treatment for insect bites, cold sores and chilblains, and can be helpful for relief of migraine. Lavender is an antiseptic and will aid the body's natural defences to fight infection acting on the spleen.
As a bath additive it is helpful in cases of rheumatism gout and sciatica.

LEMON Alkali-forming. As an antirheumatic and diuretic take 3 drops after meals. Stimulates the white corpuscles and 3-4 drops can be taken for anaemia before meals. Regulator of stomach acidity. As a gargle for sore throats 2% added to lukewarm water. 2% added to boiled water will arrest bleeding. For verrucae apply essence at night. Add to wheat germ oil for weak, brittle nails. For inflammation of the ears 10% added to lukewarm sweet almond oil. Lemon oil can also be used for food flavouring.

LEMONGRASS for use as a cleanser for oily skin when blended with base oils or water for facial rinsing or a bath additive. Opens pores.

MARJORAM is an antispasmodic and tranquilliser, especially during times of grief. A remedy for migraine, insomnia and high blood pressure and helps to disperse bruises. Relieves intestinal spasms. A powerful antispasmodic when blended with cypress and lavender.

MELISSA obtained from the herb, an antispasmodic and a tonic for the heart, uterus, nervous and digestive systems, useful for relief from nausea of a nervous origin. A low blood pressure remedy, and it will slow respiration and pulse. An antidepressant and used for allergies.

MYRRH. An expectorant and good for catarrh and especially bronchitis. An excellent remedy for mouth ulcers and mouth inflammations and is also used for external application to piles.

NEROLI (Orange Blossom). A beautiful perfume in its own right and used in many perfume preparations. Non-irritant rejuvenating agent for the skin that can be used for all skin types. A most effective anti-depressant. Also a deodorant and useful remedy for palpitations and shock.

PATCHOULI obtained from the herb and has an unusual perfume reputed to be an aphrodisiac, Helps to reduce inflammation and used in the treatment of water retention.

PEPPERMINT. Why take aspirin when you can take peppermint. 1-2 drops taken internally can work wonders in dissolving abdominal pains, digestive, menstrual etc. Also helps to alleviate migraine when taken and when a little is applied to the forehead. An effective inhalant. No better remedy for mosquito bites and similar flying pests. A MUST for your first aid cabinet. Excellent also for food flavouring and making liqueur.

PINE (Sylvestris). A mental revitaliser, an antiseptic for the respiratory system, urinary tract and liver. Antirheumatic and a useful inhalant combined with eucalyptus, lavender and thyme.

ROSEMARY obtained from the herb. Used as a rinse for the hair it stimulates the blood circulation to the scalp encouraging hair growth. If used regularly it will slightly darken the hair, An antiseptic and dandruff inhibitor and a stimulant for the circulation and the nerves. If using in the bath use in the morning not at night if you are an insomniac. A high/low blood pressure remedy because of its effect on the tension of blood vessels. Used for asthma, nervous heart, sinus problems and combined with lavender in a massage oil alleviates rheumatic pain.

SANDALWOOD, a very pleasing natural aromatic perfume obtained from the inner wood of the tree. Good for relief of chest complaints and sore throats. It is a useful oil for dry and mature skin, and can be used as a diarrhoea remedy.

THYME obtained from the flower heads and used for flatulence, fatigue, anaemia, leucorrhoea, influenza and as a general stimulant. Thyme baths are helpful for bruises, swellings and sprains, paralysis, and particularly for nervous exhaustion. Massage oil of thyme can also be used for shingles.

YLANG YLANG, a very popular oil for its perfume, obtained from the flowers of the tree. A hormone balance, general tonic and a high blood pressure remedy. Used for oily skin. A relaxant and claimed to have powerful aphrodisiac qualities! Helpful for pre-menstrual tension. Regulates cardiac and respiratory rhythm.

JASMINE. A truly exquisite perfume, and an ingredient of most exclusive perfumes. Helpful for conditions of a depressive, nervy nature. An anti-spasmodic, particularly for uterine problems.

ROSE. A lovely lingering perfume and like jasmine a touch of real luxury. Soothing for the nerves and excellent for the female reproductive system, cleansing and regulating. Gently tones the whole body. Wonderful for mature, dry and sensitive skin.

AROMATHERAPY MASSAGE OILS

The massage oils listed are those found to be most popular and helpful. If you have any special requirements or queries please write to us. The essential oils are blended in a Sweet Almond Oil base, which is an excellent oil in its own right. Wheat germ and Avocado base oils are also available.

BERGAMOT/CLARY SAGE is a beautiful fragrant combination of oils. Lifts depression and nervous tension and is a relaxant of some repute. Aids deep sound sleep if massaged into the face at night. Aids deep breathing, as bergamot clears the bronchial tubes. Do not drive after massaging with clary sage as it induces drowsiness.
This combination can also be used to prepare the tissues before an abdominal operation.

BERGAMOT/JUNIPER A delightful blend encouraging deep natural and restful breathing.
Also helpful for acne sufferers.

CLARY SAGE A very powerful relaxant, induces drowsiness and deep sound sleep. Massage into face on going to bed.
Do not drive after massaging with this combination because of its effect.

CYPRESS/NEROLI A tonic with soothing effect for broken veins.

FRANKINCENSE/JUNIPER An astringent for oily skin. Helpful for piles and catarrh.
A pleasant perfume inducing deep breathing.

FRANKINCENSE Popular for its perfume alone. A lung tonic.

GINGER A warming massage oil useful at onset of cold to induce perspiration.
Helpful for backache relief.

JUNIPER/CEDARWOOD/BERGAMOT Wonderful natural remedy for those who suffer from cystitis. Rub gently on lower abdomen. See section on concentrated essential oil of Juniper. Also for use on oily skin to stimulate the circulation and tone the skin.

NEROLI/JASMINE Beautiful facial massage for dry sensitive skin, makes you feel rejuvenated and wonderfully pampered.

SWEET FENNEL/BLACK PEPPER Aids muscle tone. For constipation, indigestion and cellulitis. Sweet Fennel is an anti-wrinkle remedy.

WHEATGERM OIL/LEMON A treatment for weak and brittle nails. Soak or massage the nails in warmed oil for 10 minutes at night.

LAVENDER/CAMOMILE Anti-allergic, soothing massage oil. Also for muscular aches after sporting activities.
LAVENDER/CAMPHOR A first aid remedy for application to injuries such as bangs and sprains, prevents swelling and bruising.

LAVENDER/CYPRESS/MARJORAM A powerful antispasmodic and varicose vein remedy.
If using over actual veins only massage VERY gently.

LAVENDER/EUCALYPTUS Massaged over the sinuses has a warming and soothing effect (not too close to the eyes). Wonderful chest remedy, and helps to increase the body's resistance to infection.

LAVENDER/GERANIUM Used for all skin types including dry eczema, and for menopausal problems. For weeping eczema see concentrated Juniper.

LAVENDER/HYSSOP/ROSEMARY Excellent for spasmodic coughs and cardiovascular disorders.

LAVENDER/LEMON Anti-rheumatic, alkali forming in action, stimulating the white blood corpuscles. Invigorating to the skin.

LAVENDER/LEMONGRASS Excellent as a cleanser for oily skin.

LAVENDER/MARJORAM/BERGAMOT Relaxant for muscle spasms and migraine sufferers.

LAVENDER/MELISSA A pleasant lemony perfume, antiallergic, antidepressant and for nausea of a nervous origin.

LAVENDER/NEROLI A beautiful perfume, non-irritant and can be used for all skin types.
One of the most effective antidepressants, deodorant, and also useful for palpitations and a relaxing massage oil.

LAVENDER/ROSEMARY One of our most popular massage combinations. This massage oil has a warming effect on the whole body and is therefore soothing and therapeutic for arthritis and rheumatic pain, and is convenient for massaging into painful fingers. A good liver tonic and remedy for migraine, colitis, catarrh, alopecia, cellulitis.
Increases the body's resistance to infection.

LAVENDER/ROSEMARY/THYME Similar effects to the lavender and rosemary combination but with the addition of Thyme it is excellent if you are feeling very tired and need a lift!
Thyme is the remedy for nervous exhaustion.

LAVENDER/SANDALWOOD Excellent for dry and sensitive skins and having a rejuvenating effect. Has antiseptic qualities and is useful for chest complaints and sore throats.
A very pleasing aromatic perfume is created by this combination.

LAVENDER/ YLANG YLANG Tonic pick-up for depression, especially pre-menstrual. Hormone balance and claimed to be an aphrodisiac! Massaged into the face at night it aids the release of nervous tension and sound sleep. Increases body's resistance to infection.

AROMATIC SUN TAN OIL This preparation has been well tried by many, with very satisfying results. The particular combination used increases the photosensitivity of the skin, while preventing the burning and drying effect of the sun and wind.

OILS FOR NATURAL BEAUTY
(Take care to keep oil out of the eyes)
Base Oils for Blending: Avocado: Sweet Almond: Wheat germ

AVOCADO OIL Like Wheat germ oil is thicker than Sweet Almond oil but because of its low viscosity it aids absorption into the skin providing proteins and vitamins, nourishing the skin.

SWEET ALMOND OIL This fine light, soothing and healing oil is excellent for general use and is also useful for removal of make-up and skin suffering from exposure to sun and wind.
WHEAT GERM OIL An anti-oxidant so keeps well and has a high vitamin E content is particularly good for dry skin leaving skin very smooth, strengthens weak and brittle nails. The skin can absorb all vegetable oils whereas mineral oils often found in cosmetics only oil the surface of the skin.

PURE ESSENTIAL OILS TO BE USED WITH THE BASE OILS AND FACIAL RINSING

Normal Skin	Geranium: Lavender: Neroli
Dry Skin	Geranium: Sandalwood: Frankincense (last two for mature skin): Fennel for the treatment of wrinkles and cellulite.
Oily Skin	Bergamot: Juniper: Cedarwood: Lemongrass: Frankincense: Ylang Ylang Geranium Helium
Inflamed or sensitive skin	Calendula: Chamomile: Lavender: Neroli
Allergies	Chamomile: Melissa
Toning the Skin	Lavender: Lemon: Peppermint (will stimulate but feels very cool when applied to the skin - keep away from the eyes): Thyme
Cleansing	Lemongrass (for oily skin): Geranium
Moisturising	Chamomile: Neroli
Circulation Stimulation	Lavender and Rosemary together
Treatment of Psoriasis	Lavender and Bergamot together
Treatment of Eczema	Dry eczema - See Lavender/Geranium
Weeping eczema	See Juniper concentrate

Acne Remedies:	Bergamot - a good antiseptic and healing agent
Camphor	A stimulant of the circulation and used for inflammation for oily acne type skin
Cedarwood	For skin eruptions, and antiseptic and relieves itching
Juniper	An antiseptic, stimulates the circulation and used for cleansing and toning the skin
Lavender	For all skin types, a skin rejuvenating agent
Sandalwood	An antiseptic and mild astringent

AROMATIC BATHS

3-4 drops of the concentrate of your choice, some essences such as sandalwood can be used more liberally. Use either for their perfume or their therapeutic effects. If the skin is very dry use avocado and wheat germ oil on their own or as a base with your favourite essence making your own bath oils.

DEODORIZING OILS

Bergamot: Clary Sage: Cypress: Eucalyptus: Lavender: Neroli: Patchouli

MOST POPULAR OILS

Perfume Oils (in the bath or for use as a perfume): Frangipani: Jasmine: Lily of the Valley. Musk and Rose Fragrance make a delightful bath blend together or used individually.

Bergamot	Refreshing
Clary Sage	A relaxant of some repute

Geranium	For all skin types
Lavender	A rejuvenating agent for the skin
Neroli	A lovely perfume
Sandalwood	For dry skin
Ylang Ylang	Soothing effect on the skin and nerves and a beautiful perfume
Juniper/Lavender/Rosemary	For tired aching feet!
Lavender/Thyme/Rosemary	When feeling exhausted

POPULAR WITH THE MEN

Black Pepper	A stimulating aphrodisiac!
Cypress	Relaxing and refreshing
Frankincense	Soothing and luxurious
Juniper	Refreshing, stimulates the circulation and ideal for skin disorders
Lemon/Thyme	Invigorates the skin
Pine	Mental revitaliser
Sandalwood	Relieves itching and inflammation

POT-POURRI

Creates a lovely lingering aroma, evoking a feeling of summer freshness all year *round*. For color and fragrance use a pot pouri mix of Peony petals, Sunflower petals, Roses Mimosa, Blue Mallow and Larkspur.

FIXATIVES
Clary Sage oil Orris Root fragrant powder Patchouli oil

POPULAR OILS
Bergamot, Clary Sage, Frangipani, Geranium, Lavender, Lemon, Lemongrass, Musk Fragrance, Patchouli, Poppy, Rose, Rosemary and Sandalwood

Recommended Book:
Pot Pourri - From Your Garden - Juniper Press

HERB PILLOW FRAGRANCES
Try one of the following oils for their soothing fragrance on a tissue on your pillow at night: Chamomile, Clary Sage, Geranium, Lavender, Lemongrass, Marjoram, Pine, Rosemary or Thyme

ROOM REFRESHERS, SPRAYS, INHALANTS etc.
Make your own room fresheners or sprays to suit your needs and moods e.g. Cypress for influenza. Bergamot, Eucalyptus, Juniper as disinfectants or perhaps Rose and Lavender.

FIRST AID:

BERGAMOT or

EUCALYPTUS — Apply directly to cold sores at onset of symptoms

CAMPHOR — For bruises, sprains, and also a strong stimulant (not to be used during pregnancy or if epileptic).

FENNEL (Sweet) * — A natural cough mixture. Mix 2/3 drops of sweet fennel oil with 1 tablespoon of honey. Dosage: 1 teaspoon to be taken as necessary.

JUNIPER — Cystitis remedy - 2 drops three times a day and take plenty of fluids.

LAVENDER	Minor burns, grazes, a general antiseptic.
MYRRH	Mouth ulcers.
NEROLI	Shock remedy.
PEPPERMINT	Very effective for headaches and digestive upsets - 1 or 2 drops in water or on sugar. Good remedy for insect bites.

One of many recommendations, Aromatherapy - The Use of Plant Essences in Healing.
by R. Lautie D.Sc./Andre Passebecq M.D. D.Ps.

If you want to know more please write to the address indicated as I have used these products and believe them to be of really good quality.

Purple Flame Aromatics,
61 Clinton Lane,
Kenilworth, CV8 1AS, Warwickshire.
Telephone (0926) 55980 (Co. Reg. No. 2533698)

Reiki Healing It's Great Mate.

Personally I had been doing the Laying on of Hands for a great number of years using spiritual healing I had been taught. I intuitively knew, and according to my clients, was very successful at being a clear channel for God's energy. When I was introduced to Reiki, I was really sceptical and half-hearted, as I could not see how it would help me too much. Curiosity got the better of me however as I saw newly certified Reiki practitioners channel energy at the high volume rates that I had only seen with experienced healers from the British Isles and the Philippines with almost lifetime of practice in the old modes of spiritual healing. After a lot of procrastination I had my initiation into Reiki through a very caring lady in Sweden and found that the symbols put into my aura and chakras (energy centres) really increased the flow of love and healing energy through my hands. It was really astonishing to find that I also had the ability and power to heal myself, which was not taught before in most of the spiritual churches I had attended.

If you can find a certified Reiki practitioner who is dedicated to the work, and most are, then you are very lucky indeed. I have seen quite a few miracles performed with the use of Reiki, like the shrinking of cancer lumps and the disappearance of major pain, vertebrae realigned in unaligned backs, broken bones mended in record time and phantom pains gone for good.

I suggest that anyone who has had a health problem looks into getting taught as not only do you learn how to place your hands on a body appropriately and learn how to energise your own body where you have pain, but also you can develop a great support group. These can be fantastic when you are at your wit's end and can't see your way clear.

Reiki (pronounced ray-key) is a Japanese word representing Universal Life Energy.

REI describes the universal limitless aspect of this energy and KI is the vital life energy.

Reiki accelerates the body's ability to heal physical ailments and opens the mind to the causes of disease and pain, promoting the joys of balance, wellness and allows the person to take responsibility for their life.

Reiki is a natural method of healing and a simple, yet powerful tool to help you take control of your life. It is not massage, and treatments are conducted fully clothed. The person giving the treatment simply places their hands in various positions for maximum energy flow around the head and body of the receiver.

Life force energy flows through the person giving the treatment to the receiver who usually receives a feeling of peace and wellbeing.

Reiki can be given in a seated position lasting up to 30 minutes working in the auric fields, or lying on a massage table lasting 1-1 ½ hours.

A Japanese scholar Dr Mikao Usui, discovered Reiki in the late 1800s, after undertaking an extensive study of the healing phenomena of history's greatest spiritual masters and leaders. He spent the rest of his life practicing Reiki and teaching people to heal with this method.

Reiki reduces stress and promotes a deep relaxation and feeling of well-being, eases pain, relieves colds, flues, headaches, burns, cuts, nausea allergies, sport injuries etc. Reiki complements medical treatments and other healing systems, reduces the side effects of drugs, and aids in the withdrawal of addictive drugs while enhancing the positive effects.

Reiki clients have experienced improved memory, creativity and learning ability and a deeper understanding of the self. It is helpful in pregnancy, the birthing process, facilitates rapid healing of broken bones and is effective on animals and plants.
It is highly recommended and there are many books now on the subject like Reiki the Healing Touch by William Rand and Living Reiki Takata's Teachings.
It is quite amazing what energy can be channelled, as the photo shows.

A student of Reiki Master, Faye Matthews, took this next photo while she was giving a Reiki initiation to another student. Faye practices The Usui System and Jin Kei Do. 07 3354 1619 www.Reiki-lifeunlimited.com.

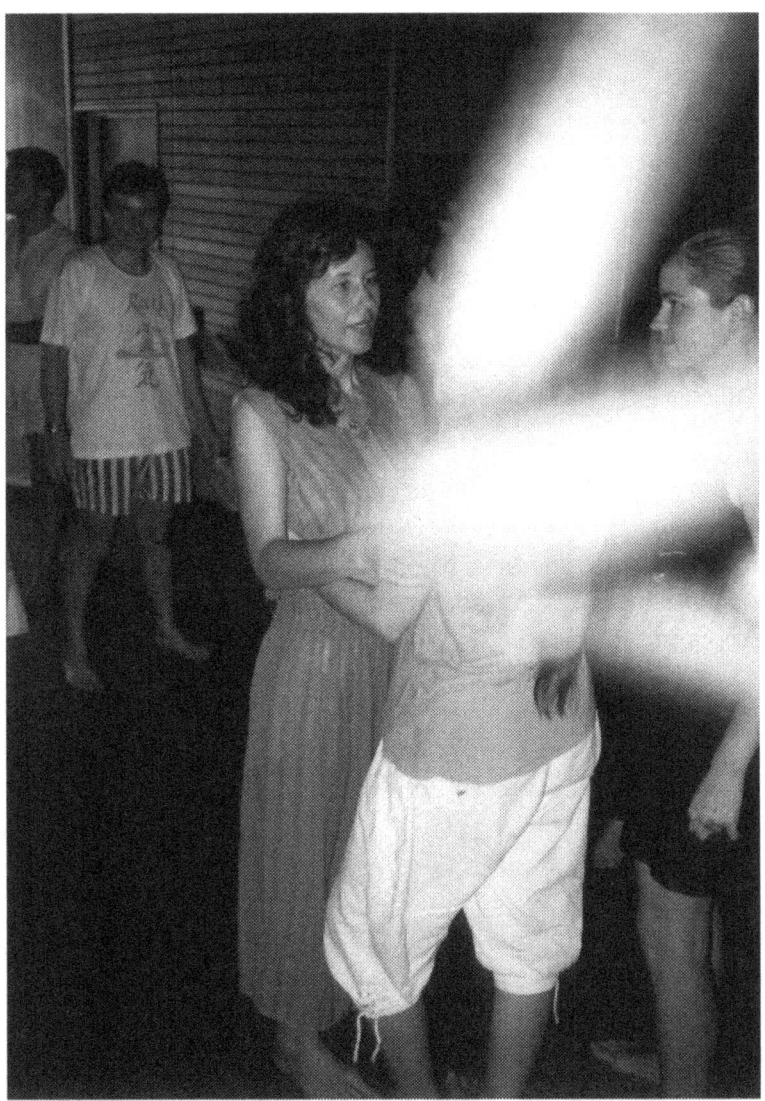

I have a manual on Reiki One where it describes what Reiki is and photos on where to place the hands, etc., so one can practice before initiation. www.healingconnection.com.au

Natural Pain Relievers

Hot baths in Epsom salts as hot as you can stand for 20 - 30 minutes will relieve swelling and stress in muscles and back /stress problems. Tired /sore feet in a bucket of warm water with three drops of Tea Tree Oil and hand full of Epsom salts.

Sauna and spa baths to help get the toxins out and perspire through the skin.

Colonics (irrigations) to wash out the toxins in the intestines and colon. A series of at least three close together within five days works best.

Medical Magnets to change the polarity of the disease. These magnets are really strong.

Castor oil packs. Cold pressed castor oil put onto a cotton pad as warm as the sore spot can handle with a heat pack on it for at least 20-30 minutes for seven days night and morning. (not an open wound) Stop for five days and then continue as before for two more sessions of seven and five days. There have been great results but it can get a bit messy. Edgar Casey the sleeping prophet remedy.

Red cabbage juice for radioactivity and ulcers.

Cranberry juice and or colloidal silver for bladder infections.

Wheat grass juice can be grown and juiced as blood cleansers and to get vital nutrients.

Barley grass for those intolerant of wheat grass as a blood cleanser and essential nutrients.

Acidophilus / bifidus for stomach upsets. Refrigerated is best.

Royal jelly for memory, balancing the hormones and premature ejaculation.

Aromatherapy oils to help with the emotional and physical bodies and environmental needs.

Herbs like Garlic are good antibiotics. Body test, check for compatibility.

Talk to your herbalist first as there are **some herbs that should not be used as remedies without expert help**.

A small list of these is Borage, Broom, Chaparral, Coltsfoot, Comfrey, Foxglove, Pennyroyal, Pokeweed, Rue, Sassafras and potential danger with some Aloe Vera internally.

Also in excessive amounts Ephedra, Juniper and Licorice.

Negative ioniser in a polluted or smog area does wonders for the air we breathe as it seems to attach to the pollen and smog which falls to the ground leaving the air smelling like one walking near a waterfall.

Cracked heals and rough skin on feet. One part water, one part glycerine, one part medical methylated spirits and mix and apply topically on skin when dry or at night.

A positive frame of mind will beat anything! While attending an Alfa Dynamics seminar the instructor told us that a man in New York who had been positive all his life agreed to be injected with cancer cells for a lot of money. The next day the cancer cells were dead, so know that a positive frame of mind is very important. From then on class members were instructed to say to themselves that they would not join the mass thinking and would refuse to get the flu again and it worked for all of those who reinforced this belief.

Computer Radiation, Microwaves

Have these checked for low frequency radiation using a Gauss meter and use a filter screen to stop computer radiation and to ground harmful radiation. Remember the cheap computer may not be cheap in the long run if it affects your health.

If you want to see the effects microwaves have on food then look up on Kirlian photography of all the different types of food. It has been proven to me beyond doubt that the food cooked in a microwave reduced the vitamin and energy value of the food. These things leak radiation and there is research done now which indicate microwaved food causes cancer-type effects on the blood, lowers haemoglobin values, and leads to degeneration.

It seems that the electrical activity of cells in raw food will enhance the vitality and improve the whole digestive process.

Organic food corona radiations show up as 50 per cent greater than non-organic.

Tinned vegetables show weak and broken energy fields while a group of vegetables grew weaker over the two to three weeks that they were stored which goes to show that fresh is best.

Microwaving seemed to reduce brightness and greatly disorganise the corona field. ie. Life force of the vegetable.

Using the same food comparing vitality after cooking conventionally and with a microwave the conventional food has always had a better vitality rate when checked with the SE-5 by a large margin.

Dr Fujimoto from Castle Hospital Wellness Program talks about dioxins and how bad they are for us. Heating food in fat, high heat, foam containers and plastics releases dioxins into the food and ultimately into the cells of the body. If you must use the microwave at least use corning ware or ceramic containers. This goes for heating TV dinners too.

A fan forced glass/Pyrex counter top oven where the food is cooked in its own juices at almost the same speed as a microwave works the best and is the healthiest so far.

The Refrigerator

Old refrigerators need to be checked by an independent person for leakage of freeon gas, as they can leak freeon gas into the food and affect your immune system, leaving you a very sick puppy. If it is leaking, please don't sell it to someone else, as you will be giving some unsuspecting person a disease too. HAVE IT DESTROYED AND IF YOU DUMP IT, TAKE THE FRONT DOOR OFF SO NO CHILD OR ANIMAL GETS LOCKED IN IT AND DIES.

Music.

Noise can put your whole body out of synchronicity if you are not careful to avoid the harsh sounds of Rap and Heavy metal etc. and stay with soft gentle music of the masters like Beethoven, etc. to help heal. There are many good new age tapes now on the market. Move away from, or put buffers around your home to muffle the noise level coming from passing traffic as this puts your body into stress at least subconsciously if not consciously. If you do have to be in places with lots of noise visit your local music store and see if you can get something like Steven Halpin's Spectrum Suite radio cassette or CD. With a Walkman and headset you will be able to control the environment a little better. There are also some really good CD/cassette tapes available now in self-hypnosis and machines which play nature sounds to block out the traffic noises so you can get a better sleep. Earplugs can be good too block out noise but make sure your environment is safe first.

Warning; Do not believe everything the manufacturers are saying about how the millions of words of subliminal messages in the music background are good for you especially if they cannot tell you what all the messages are or give you a copy of them. They may work for some, however, all they do for many people is make them very irritable and aggressive. I like to see where a person is at and know if it has worked for them, walking their path or just out selling another gimmick. I still have not found one tape with subliminal messages that works for me and on testing with kinesiology and the SE-5 the indications are to leave the subliminal messages alone as I do not know what is programmed into my head without my permission.

Toning

I believe toning, by a skilled practitioner to be very good and I have seen some new technology where a computer analyses your voice then plays back various sounds or tones to give you the vibrations you are missing. I have heard the results are astonishing. In case you do not know, sound will also produce a vibration close to color. In days gone by, there were also many older healers who used a pendulum to find out what colour suited the affliction. This color was laid over the diseased part of the body or the healer would mentally place that color into the diseased organ with great results I might add.

COLOR

Color is important to healing so if you are wearing drab colors it's time to change and have a personal color analysis done by a color therapist to see what colours suit you and what don't. Correct colors enhance your aura and other colors draw your energy power out.

Let me explain the basic colors in the colors of the rainbow as I understand it. In the beginning for primitive man there was the light of day in which man hunted or was hunted and for survival at night when it was dark. He rested as it was either dark blue or black. As he couldn't see he rested up in a tree or a cave until morning action came about again. Light was action, dark blue was rest time and black was the absence of light and was normally feared because one couldn't see the predators which was dangerous. Needless to say if one was stalking another to hurt or kill and wore black clothing, he would be doing this to shut out the light (God's light) so he would not have to feel that this was wrong.

Black is the absence of color, the end beyond which there is nothing more. It represents renunciation, the ultimate surrender or relinquishment. Someone who wears a lot of black usually wants subconsciously to renounce everything against the existing state in which he feels that nothing is as he feels it should be. It is amazing that when I used to wear black how I was able to draw negative situations to me although I was also able to express anger freely at the world. Don't rock my boat or you will be hurt badly. My teenage years and tough as hell.

White represents the day, the spiritual light of God. When a prism is put under a white light it splits the light into the colors of the rainbow. It is therefore very healing to visualise bringing a white light down from your source, wherever that may be depending on your religion or upbringing, and cover a diseased or in need person with that white light. Also to fill your own being like a bottle full of water. To me this is like a signpost saying to God, Universal energies, Great Mysteries, whatever you may call it, that this person needs help, so please help him.

When people pray in a prayer circle for someone at a church or during a meditation group, I clairvoyantly see and clairsentiantly sense a great ball of white light going from the circle of people to the afflicted person. The person then has the ability to use the energy to get well or it will stay in the aura until he needs it once the decision has been made to either stay or go Home. Heaven if you prefer.

Let's digress for a minute.

Remember we are all **energy piranhas** when we are unwell or have a dis-ease. Every time I mention this in a seminar I hear a lot of indignation, so read this next bit carefully, as I am only a two-finger typist and will not repeat it unless I need to.

When a person is in hospital with a major dis-ease or having an operation and is resting up, he just wants to be alone in their pain as he is normally groggy and any noise is magnified, so who needs visitors. At that time all the friends, aunts, uncles and acquaintances turn up, bringing lots of flowers and gifts and sit like ghouls around the bed and whisper about their aches and pains. Then they go home saying that the patient didn't even talk to them and you would think they had put in a large day of work as they are so tired. THEY HAVE JUST GIVEN THEIR ENERGY TO THE PATIENT TO USE TO GET WELL. So did the flowers. You may notice the sicker a person is the quicker the flowers die.

The same thing happens while driving a car, after a good night out on the town. On the drive home, what happens? Generally everyone in the car falls asleep even though they may be charged up before they left and the driver usually complains that no one stays awake to talk to him. You have all just willingly given your energy to keep alive, as the driver needs your energy to stay awake and get you all home safely.

Another good example of this is where a man who has a lot of little girls in his family will feel the need to go out with the boys now and again to top up his energy tanks as little children can really drain one if they are not happy. For mothers and fathers it is extremely important to leave the children with someone safe for at least a couple of days a month to re- energise the light levels of themselves.

Ask any practiced clairvoyant and they will tell you that this is so.

If you are around someone who is sick or depressed, then you must take time out for yourself. The person you are with may be drawing too much of your energy and you may need to replenish it by going out to be with someone of your own sex to top up the energy tanks. I am not talking sexually here, just friendship.

Gray is a neutral color and is uncommitted, wants to wall everything off, unwilling to take part in life and insulating self from direct participation by only dealing with what they must mechanically and artificially. A lifeless calm.

Brown is to me unless mixed with other colors, is a lack of color in one's life, and the need to get back to the earth. The nondescript, boring life lacking the vibrancy of joy and intimacy. Little prospect of physical security and contentment ahead of them.

Red is a physical color and has a slow vibration. People who are very physical will use red to calm the physical body when in pain or raise their sexual drive as red has a stimulating effect on the nervous system. Blood pressure increases respiration rate and heartbeat both speed up while wearing red. Notice how often if ladies want to attract a man they put on a really slinky red dress. Great mate! Red is therefore exciting in its stimulating effect on the nervous system, especially on the sympathetic branch of the autonomic nervous system and is the expression of the vital force, the will to win, intensity of living and fullness of experience. Lack of red in the system usually indicates there is irritability, lack of vitality and seeking protection.

When you mentally surround and infuse your mind with red you will find your body calm and be much less stiff and rigid.

Orange is the color of the emotions and a person wearing a lot of orange is usually trying to calm the emotions. Notice a lot of successful restaurants use orange combined with yellow to calm the emotions and intellect so you will enjoy your relaxed meal more and buy more food. When you mentally surround yourself with orange you will find yourself calming and stilling your emotions.

Yellow is the brightest of the colors and corresponds to the warmth of sunlight when the light has come to the planet, to cheerfulness and a happy spirit, release of burdens, problems and restrictions. Yellow has the effect of calming the intellect so you will find yellow usually on the walls of a bedroom of a person who is highly intellectual. Maybe a lemon shade. Don't believe me, then check out the local universities. We did. It was fun. When you mentally surround yourself in a yellow color it has the effect of calming the mind chatter.

Green represents in ancient mythology peace, healing and harmony. A lot of hospitals have their staff dressed in green. The old ideas of looking at something green when stressed would have a soothing calmness to it. In shooting I was taught that when the eyes got blurry from too much concentration, look at something green over your right shoulder and the vision would right itself within a few seconds. Persons wearing green want to increase their certainty in their own value or pride and self worth.

Blue represents love, peace and calm and has a pacifying effect on the nervous system so that blood pressure, respiration rate and pulse are all reduced. The need for this color increases emotional tranquillity, peace, harmony and contentment or in the psychological need for rest and recuperation. Remember the old songs Love is Blue, Blue Bird of Happiness, etc.

Indigo or purple This color is a spiritual color and until recently was reserved for royalty or the church alter and those high up on the ladder in the churches called Cardinals and Popes and suchlike. It was meant to represent a person of high integrity who has given up their free will to work for God or the people with not too much of a reward to themselves. The people kept royalty by paying them taxes to protect and manage all the affairs of the kingdom. The priests were to manage all the spiritual affairs of the people like births, deaths and marriages and when called for to help the sick and needy, with an occasional exorcism thrown in for good measure.

In my opinion many seem to have failed their position and the test given them by God or the universe, and now chase the almighty dollar and greed.

Now don't get me wrong, I am not against religion in any way, but how would you feel if you had children in another country, and you saw half of them starving and the other half building beautiful buildings to commemorate you giving them birth and life. Hoping it would please you to grant them favours and encourages you (God) and new church members to visit them in their wonderful new buildings. What would you do? I have seen more miracles by those walking their talk then those talking their walk.

Not only that but exorcism and spiritual releasement was an exclusive job for the church and thankfully is coming back into the work of the churches once more. In Eastern religions this has never stopped. After people die the priests get together and call the soul of the deceased person and tell him to forgive himself and go home to the light. They are told they have been forgiven, to let go control on those they have left behind, that God will not punish them, but they may have to judge themselves knowing and having all knowledge of the facts, and to leave this plain of existence. This still occurs today behind closed doors, and was in western religions too until those in charge chased power and greed instead of helping the flock.

This is not to be feared just because it cannot be seen or sensed by most untrained people. I always look at the end result and if what is written here is a whole load of garbage to you, that's OK by me because maybe it does not affect you. Maybe it's imagination but I have seen so many people's lives improve dramatically after doing some spiritual releasement work with them, and I know it works. This does not mean that people should go on a witch hunt and blame their whole life on negative entities taking charge of their lives. Whenever I have a client who has a family dis-ease recurring through the generations then there is a good possibility that there is a family entity scared to go into the light and is drawing energy from and trying to manipulate those on earth. Anyone who is sensitive will take on the disease of the deceased and will manifest or react in this way just about immediately.

The ancient rituals of soul releasement were nearly all forgotten but are now being retaught by spiritual churches and beautiful people like Dr Edith Fiore Ph. D. of Squaw Valley in California in her book The Unquiet Dead. Dr William Baldwin DDS Ph.D and his wife Judith did enormous amounts of research and confirmed for me on the physical level what I already knew and saw in Spirit.

Dr William Baldwin's book on Regressional Therapy and Spirit Releasement Therapy Technique manual can be obtained from PO Box 4061 Enterprise Florida 32725 USA.
The cost is approximately $50. Bill also runs courses for professionals in this work all over the world. Other books on this are Thirty Years Among the Dead by Dr Carl Wickland, The Tibetan Book Of The Dead and the Egyptian Book Of The Dead.

Mrs. Bea Harper also does spiritual releasement work at a distance from a photograph or handwriting of the person for a nominal cost. She will write back to you to tell you what stray energies she picks up in your aura, car, house or the place you work in.
This lady has been a miracle worker for me and for clients who I have recommended to write to her. The results are nothing short of miraculous. What have you got to lose except unhappiness and unwanted HITCHIKERS? The following is the sheet she sends out explaining her work after she has completed the work.

THE HEALING MINISTRY OF RELEASE
Mark 16:17
The work you requested has been completed. This sheet contains general information so that you may better understand. The term D.E. is used for Discarnate Entity. This simply means a consciousness that has left its body through death and is now an energy form, invisible to us. These D.E.s are earthbound, they do not wish to

leave and go on in their progression because they are emotionally attached to their former habits. They enter or attach themselves to a living person at the first opportunity, usually in order to enjoy their habits vicariously. Sometimes the entry is accidental and they find themselves locked in and unable to leave. Entrance is made through a break or crack in the aura, and they may be found inside the physical (Possession), Inside the aura, or attached outside the aura which is the area of least influence. There are also some D.E.s that stay due to fear of hell and eternal damnation as taught in childhood.

Each person is checked for D.E.s, Possession, Mind Control, Hex, Spell, Curse or Implant. If any of these are present, it is explained individually. We try to find if any entrance was made at birth. The most common way they enter is through **mind-expanding drugs or alcohol**, but they can also come in when one is deeply under an anaesthetic or momentarily unconscious from a blow or fall. Strong emotional outbursts like anger can draw them. At such times, being beside yourself with rage or out of your mind are quite true. Therefore we are urged to practice control of thoughts and feelings. Trying to contact the next plane of existence through a ouija board or automatic writing is dangerous as it usually attracts the lower entities.

A new service has been added. We now check for Supra-physical shells from a person's own previous life. Usually these disintegrate between lives, but if the energy put into the problem was strong enough, it remains animated and is magnetically drawn to the body at birth. Dennis Kelsey and Joan Grant explain this in their book Many Lifetimes. We find these can be dissolved and transmuted by the Angels of the Violet Flame.

In the analysis, your original handwriting or picture is placed under a chart over an open bible. We contact your High Self and Guardian Angel for the information and permission. Personality measurements are taken before and after the release to determine where the D.E. influence was greatest. A numbered scale is used, but to keep it simple we say below and above average or average.

Average is for metaphysical students or seekers of truth. Inner stress measures the amount of pressure or opposition between the real self and the D.E.s fighting for control. We also check for blocks between the high self and consciousness. The actual Release is done IN THE NAME OF JESUS CHRIST. We have trained helpers and angels on the inner planes that lead the entities off to the plane where they belong so they cannot attach to others. The home is also cleared of stray D.E.s or those left by former tenants, also the car that is sometimes invaded.

After a release, the aura is sealed in a ring of golden-white light, and the spots where the D.E.s were attached are drained and filled with love and energy. But the seal can still be broken if one continues in his old habits or fails to protect himself properly. TO PROTECT YOURSELF, visualise and FEEL a tube of White Christ Light around the body, about 3 feet out. You are literally wrapping yourself in a force field impenetrable by the dark forces. Say firmly, I STAND IN THE CHRIST LIGHT. I AM ALWAYS PROTECTED AND MY AURA IS SEALED FROM ANY NEGATIVE FORCE. Do this especially before sleep and before leaving the house in the morning.

One may notice a definite change or reaction within 48 hours after a release. One may experience severe headache, nausea, or crying spells if infiltration was deep. It usually takes from 30 to 90 days for the inner bodies to return to a normal pattern. This is because the D.E.s leave debris that must be purged. It takes time, especially if they have been there long, with certain habits and patterns established. Restoration is like reprogramming a computer and is helped by prayer, meditation, and affirmations on one's own part or for a loved one. Remember, one must be willing to change himself, his thoughts and habits, for a release to effect permanent change.

Suggested donation: $55 each. $30 for rechecks.

In any kind of healing, it is important to FORGIVE. Take time to forgive everyone who comes to mind. Past or present, and

forgive yourself for every mistake or guilty feeling. **Repeat with feeling I FORGIVE OTHERS AND I FORGIVE MYSELF. GOD FORGIVES ME AND I AM FREE.**

For those of you who think this is a load of bull look at the following police photograph taken shortly after Patrick McGann drowned and was published in the New Zealand Post. He has since gone into the light as he has found his way home. Rest In Peace.

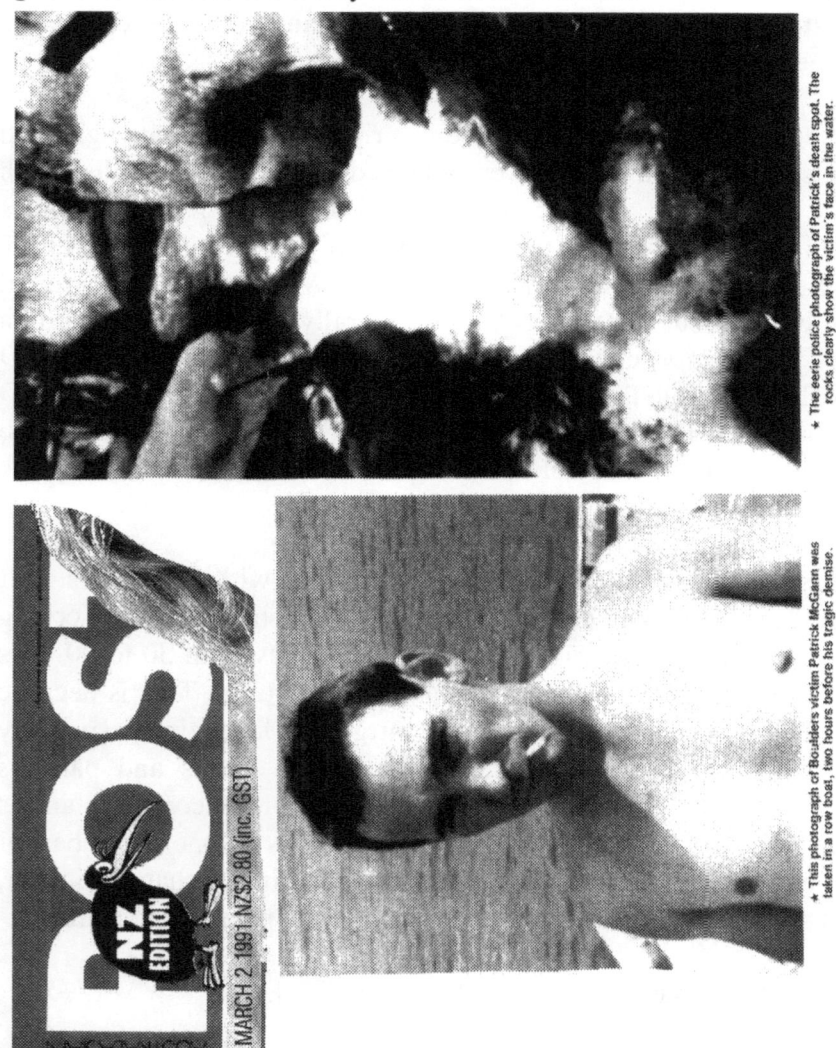

+ The eerie police photograph of Patrick's death spot. The rocks clearly show the victim's face in the water.

+ This photograph of Boulders victim Patrick McGann was taken in a row boat, two hours before his tragic demise.

Back to Aura colors

Violet has a mystical, fairyland quality to it. It can mean identification as an intimate, erotic blending or it can lead to intuitive and sensitive deep understanding of being closer to your source, wherever that may be.

In ancient times the coat of many colors was all the colors of the rainbow and to be awarded this coat meant that you had attained self-mastery, and this was a high award.

RED	when you calmed the body using red.
ORANGE	you calmed the emotions using orange.
YELLOW	stilled the mind using yellow.
GREEN	when you calmed your body mind with all of these colors, you would find peace which was green.
BLUE	you found peace you would then find love in your life and that color is blue
INDIGO	you found love in your life and you would become spiritual or want to help others, which is represented by a purple colour in the Aura.
VIOLET	this color is nearly back to red again or centered within on the higher levels. Remember the old biblical drawings of blessed masters and the clear color round the head tinged with violet.

When you became balanced with all the colors and you were a spiritual master in ancient times you had a direct HOT LINE to God. You were at peace with all beings and things knowing that God was in charge and the self would get out of the way and just BE so life could BE as it was meant to BE.

The Luscher Color Test book by Dr Max Luscher published by Washington Square Press is a really inexpensive little book that does a great analysis on color and your personality.

This is how some clairvoyants see and perceive what the colors mean. Remember if you ever have a reading from a clairvoyant, to read you they have to read through their own aura. Just as you must see through your own aura to perceive another's. The clearer your own aura, the clearer, more accurate the reading.

Red Family

Cherry	Courage, leadership, disciplined, aggressive
Fire Red	Emotional person, healing energies
Scarlet	Sensuous, temperamental
Red/Gray/Black	Confused
Magenta	Strong character
Melon	Great power, strength, honesty

Orange Family

Orange	Creative force, strong life force
Orange/Red	Magnetic healing qualities
Deep Bright Orange	Pride, egotistical

Yellow Family

Canary	Sunshine spirit
Golden Yellow	Intelligence
Lemon	Cheerful, peaceful, joy, happiness
Corn	Freedom of mind, pleasure seeker
Dark Yellow	Intellect
Pale Yellow	Spirituality, wisdom, and metaphysical development
Buff	Good reason, judgment, and perception
Eggshell	Faithful, love, truthful

Green Family

Apple Green	Prosperity, abundance
Pale Apple Green	Healer

Dark Green	Active life
Emerald Green	Creativity, versatility, ingenuity, adaptability
Nile Green	Restless, disappointed
Pale Green	Sympathy for others

Blue Family

Blue	Inspiration, intelligence
Pale Medium Blue	Peace within self
Darker Medium Blue	Frustrated by people around you
Sky Blue	Truth, spirit, purity, devotion
Indigo Blue	Inclined to study metaphysical subjects
Blue/Brown	Religiously inclined but selfish
Peacock Blue	Repose, self love, large ego

AURA POSITIVE COLORS
Pink/Lavender Family

Pink	Enduring love
Deep Pink	Domestic love, devotion, love of humankind
Salmon Pink	Love of worldly things
Heliotropes	Very sad, serious, lonely, individuality
Mauve	Spiritual love
Lavender	Gentleness, sober, great penetration
Pale Lavender	High spiritual aspirations
Lilac	Sweet character but impulsive

Purple Family

Purple	Aristocratic, worldly ambitious, great teacher, artist, composer seeking fame and honor
Deeper Purple	Great dignity and an earned self-respect
Deep Purple	High spiritual development, holy love, divine radiance.

Gray Family

| Pale Gray | Clairvoyance |
| Pearl Gray | Shy but refined, recognises spirit |

John Chamberlin

White Family
White   Purity, perfection, and light of goodness

Gold Family
Gold   Great wisdom channelled from higher
                           realms

Silver Family
Silver   Protection around you from higher realms

NEGATIVE COLOURS Understand but don't dwell on these
                           negative aspects.

Reds
Blood Red   Envy, revenge, hates
Claret Red   Suspicious mood, distrustful
Crimson Red   Immoral person, low taste and desire
Red, Deep Burnished   Very destructive, fearful
Dull Red   Animalistic
Light Crimson   Sensual, leadership with destructive bent
Ugly Crimson   Anger

Oranges
Muddy Orange   Out of sorts
Orange/Brown   Low intellect

Yellows
Yellow/Greenish/Gray   Jealousy
Yellow/Brown   Discontented
Yellow -- Watery   Foolish

Greens
Dull Green   Jealousy, anger
Olive Green   Treachery, deceit, unfaithful
Ivy Green (Dark)   Intense selfishness
Muddy Green   Fickle, selfish

Blues
Ugly Peacock Blue   Vanity, pride, tremendous ego

Whites/Gray

Ashy White	Nervous
Bright Gray	Selfish
Dull Gray	Fearful
Deep Gray	Depression

Browns

Brown	Greed, cowardice, dangerous thoughts, very destructive deep hatred.
Brown/Red Ashes	Jealousy
Seal Brown	Very cold nature

Blacks

Black	Deep, deep hatred, malice, revenge, capable of murder
Black	Despair, untruthful, deceitful
Reddish Black	Hatred, malice
Black Crimson	Revenge
Blackish Green	Treacherous

Color Healing can also be very good with a little knowledge of where to place different colors or crystals on the different energy centers, or if you live in the eastern world chakras.

COLOR IMAGE

DRESS COLORS CAN HAVE A VERY PROFOUND EFFECT ON ONE'S LIFE, AND HOW OTHERS REACT TO THEM.
The following has been prepared for you to realise what the COLOR experts say about how colors affect you, your thinking, and how your energy presents itself. My seminars called Going Beyond Seminars for business were great fun picking several people out of the group to dress up in different clothes to show people how they presented using different colors, and how dress sense and color could affect the end result of asking for the order subconsciously.

Personal style begins with color harmony, creating a harmony of colors that enhance hair, eye and skin colors that are individually unique. Personal palettes are hand selected according to a precise computer assisted analysis of the **HUE** (color family), **VALUE** (lightness or darkness) and **CHROMA** (brightness) from hair, eye and skin numeric coded data.

When you wear your best colors you express a confidence and a harmony of natural beauty that's yours alone. The computer scans all colors to identify the most flattering color harmonies that give greatest beauty and impression, and your personal palette represents the following hues:

Your colours and tones convey the following messages and images:

1. Skin Emphasises
Personal skin colors are unique, and when worn give you an appearance of warmth because all skin comes from the hues, yellow, yellow - red, or red. Skin tones have a warm Yin (Feminine) character.

2. Hair Emphasises
Hair colors are an effective form of influence in communicating a very self confident image. They highlight, draw attention to and enrich your unique hair color.

3. Eye Emphasises
Your eye colors will attract attention to your eyes. They convey an image of a peaceful, calm disposition, therefore they are good colors for communication because they project an approachable feeling and friendly, comfortable mood, establishing rapport.

Combined with skin and hair colors they create your signature colors, an individual unique combination executing a statement of your unique colouring.

4. Your Reds

Vibrant and electrifying, a color highly charged with emotion, able to speed the pulse rate. Red gets a forceful emotional message across. It has zest, excitement and power. Red is the hue on the top of the rainbow and it stays on top. It is associated with energy, winners, achievers, intense, extrovert, vitality, the language of love, sexy, passionate and absolutely feminine as a bouquet of red roses. Your reds will complement and flatter your skin tone, also rejuvenate and brighten your complexion.

6. Your Wine Reds

These colors are rich, elegant and refined, from the same family of Yang (masculine) reds, carrying more authority, command, dignity and weight of character to them.

6. Your Pinks

A softened tint of red, subdued, toned down and subtle in warmth, emotion and charm.

7.Your Purples

Convey an image of refinement and elegance. They are rich, regal, the insignia of royalty, supremely authoritative, powerful or passionate. The color of the creative and artistic. They can be tranquil, quiet, cool, refined in manner or mood, polished, well bred, a color of excellence and good taste.

8.Your Blues

The most powerful of all colors, easy to wear, calms, peaceful, quiet, restful and serene. They are contrasting colors. Navies project a conservative, reliable, trustworthy image and an excellent background for other colors. Brighter blues can be mixed for many exciting color combinations.

9.Your Blue Greens

Soothing and ocean fresh, greens can have a connotation of energy, exciting liveliness, nature refreshing, spring like. Made up of yellow and blue, it is balance. Nature's greens promote a message of rest, peace, coolness and calmness. Green is the color of Spring and is the olive green branch symbolic of hope and a new beginning. Green communicates an image of growth and self-improvement.

10. Your Yellow Reds
A fun, friendly, happy color, connotations of being modern, daring, young, exciting, unique, flashy and not boring.

11. Your Browns
Rich and spicy, conveying a message of warmth, quality, harmony, down-to-earth, earthy. It is the color associated with stability, reliability, and a character of substance. Dark brown can be as authoritative as black and convey authority.

12. Your Yellow
Happy, lively and positive. Wearing yellow is like wearing a bit of sunshine, it's uplifting, warm and exciting.

13. Your Gray
Communicated understated authority, ultimate conservatism and neutrality, serious, mature, dignified, strong, having enduring stability.

14. Your Black
Message of sophistication and expensive connotations of mystery and sexiness. In business clothing it appears stark, severe, and yet authoritative, with reassuring background. Message of responsibility and efficiency.

15. Your Whites
Evoking attention, recall of youth, freshness and simplicity. It can look joyful, or elegantly sophisticated. It reflects light and will enhance the brilliance of any color that you will wear it with.

16. Combinations

Analogous Colors	closely related hues.
Monochromatic colors	one hue family, vary shades and tints of hues.
Complementary	colors opposite on the colour wheel, create contrast and strong attraction.
Authoritative	wear the darkest colors in the palette.
Friendly	wear the brightest colors in the palette.
Romantic	wear the light colors in the palette.

17. Create a more flattering silhouette

Use color with flair and influence to shape the figure you want and direct the eye to focus attention where you want it.

To appear taller, minimise lower areas. Color can minimise a fuller upper figure and take years off your appearance.

Color has the power to do so much

Use color to cheer you up, or change your mood. Color invokes a positive mood from others too.

Use and balance of color

Always use irregular amounts of color, which are pleasing to the eye and will keep you from fading away. Come alive with a touch of color pizzazz using varying ratios.

Etheric Bodies / Chakras /Energy Centers

We have many, many energy centers all over our bodies, usually behind every joint but there are seven main centers located as per next diagram by the red, orange, yellow, green, blue, indigo, violet dots.

The red one is the coarsest energy and also the closest to the earth with each center going up the body becomes finer and with a faster flow. The finest energy center is at the top of the head where we usually get our messages from God or guidance. According to the original East Indian traditions the main etheric energies are similar to figure in the drawing called Etheric Energies.

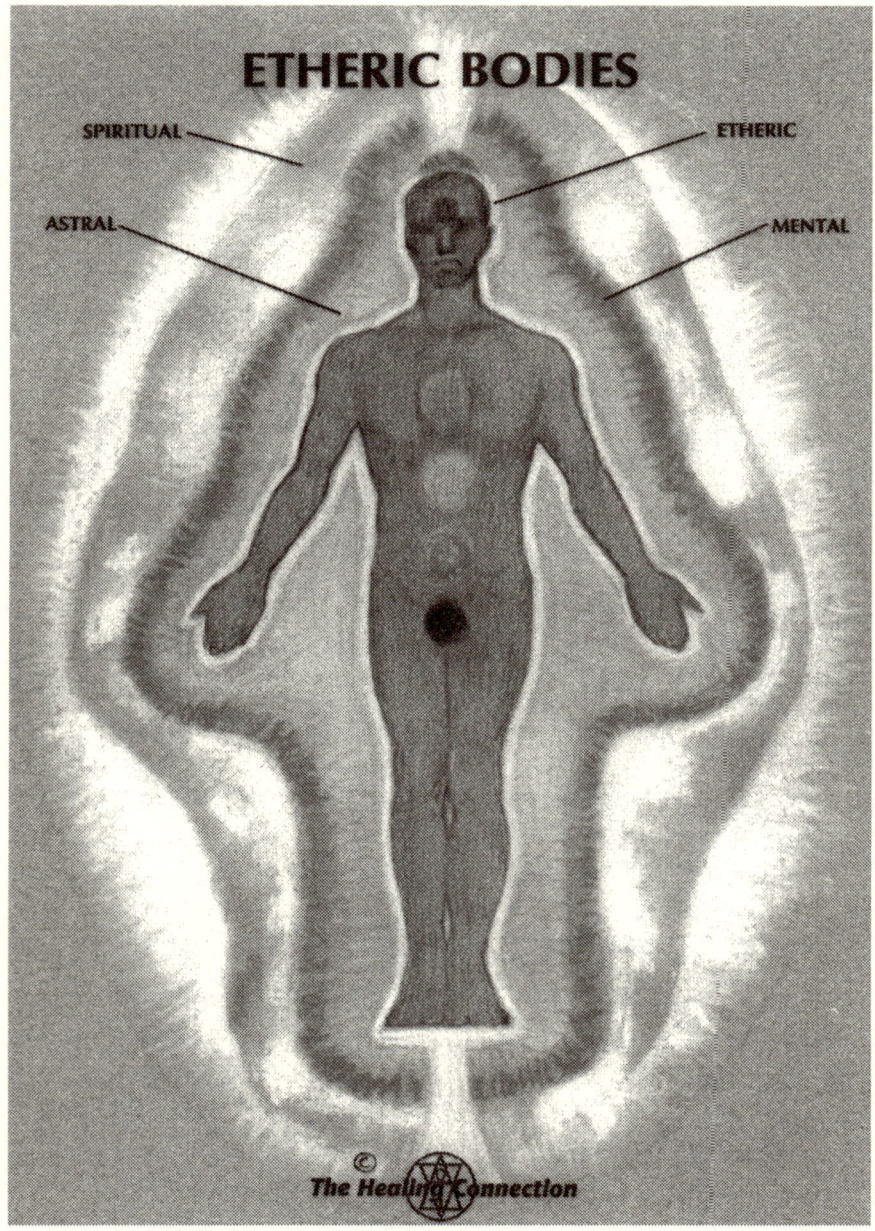

ETHERIC BODIES

SPIRITUAL

ETHERIC

ASTRAL

MENTAL

The Healing Connection

These etheric bodies can be seen with practice from your peripheral vision and there are several good books on the subject. However, I recommend a class in it as one can see better with several teachers around who are naturally visionary.

The etheric body is up to 1/2 an inch to an inch close to the body depending on how tired the person is.

This body is best seen if you let your eyes go out of focus when the subject is sitting on a stool up against a white wall with a red lamp or light bulb on the floor about three feet away at night.

The astral body is the next one out and this is the body we travel in to send love or anger to another or obtain knowledge by astral travelling when we sleep or go into trance.

The next body is the mental body that if we are positive will control the energies from the universe to give us good health and stop psychic interference.

The spiritual body controls all the bodies and is influenced by pre-patterning that we choose to have on us for this lifetime. Planets, tides and astrology influences the bodies also.

ENERGY CENTERS/MERIDIANS

The energy centers as I prefer to call them get finer and finer in energy and spin faster as they go up your body. It's almost as though we are, as I like to think, split off from God's energy/spark like little Gods/Goddesses in the making. Like our children are copies of us and like a light switch we have to be grounded to have our energy here on this planet. Our bodies are the final manifestation on this planet of God's energy coming to have our earthly experience. We refine ourselves and go back to the mother/father God to sit on the right hand of the Father/Mother to let them know what we learnt. Therefore the lowest chakra is the slowest. The final manifestation of Spirit /Soul connecting to this planet Earth.

Book The Chakras by Leadbeater shows colour plates of the centers.

These chakras actually correspond to the colors of the rainbow with the courser or the base chakra situated at the base of the spine.

This is known as the root chakra and under normal health is the color RED.

First Chakra is color red, responds to the note of C, Element of earth, Adrenal gland, Etheric energy body, Planet of Saturn and Earth.

Relates to the earth, grounding, and center of physical energy and vitality.

Balancing of this chakra can ease hidden fears, disorientation and inability to focus.

Unbalanced shows lack of confidence, lack of achieving goals, inhibition, self destructive, or suicidal, anxiety and stress.

Second Chakra located at the stomach button area and is color orange, responds to note of D, Element of water, ovaries, testicles, glands, sense of taste, mental, emotional energy body, planet moon. Relates to fluidity, friendliness, creativity, sexuality, emotions, intuition, and intimacy.

Sense of self worth, confidence in one's creative ability and the ability to relate to others in an open and friendly way. Diseases are related to internalised anger and are relieved by balancing.

Balanced energy is friendliness, optimistic, concern for others, sense of belonging, creative initiative, clairsentient, attuned to own feelings sense of humor and intimacy.

Unbalanced is shy, timid, immobilised by fear, overly sensitive, self negating, resentful buried emotions, guilt, distrustful or emotionally explosive, aggressive, frustrated, overly ambitious, manipulative, caught up in illusion, self serving.

Third Chakra located at diaphragm area is a yellow colour, Note of G, Element of fire, gland of pancreas and adrenals, affects sense of sight, energy of mental body, planet of Mars and Sun.

Qualities of personal power and authority. When open you will find your personal purpose or work that brings you joy and fulfilment. Radiates warmth, acceptance, relaxation and builds a positive self image. Rules digestion and mind. Balancing this Chakra helps integrate emotions around mother and getting in touch with one's feminine self.

Balanced energy is outgoing, cheerful, self-respecting, with a strong sense of personal power. Personal will align with divine will. Skilful, intelligent, relaxed, spontaneous expressive.

Unbalanced energy is depressed, lack of confidence, always worrying about what others will think, and belief of others' control, poor digestion, afraid of living alone **or** judgmental, workaholic, perfectionist, overly intellectual, may need drugs to relax, superiority complex fluctuates with inferiority complex.

Fourth Chakra is located on the heart area. Is the colour green, note of G, Element of air, Gland is thymus, touch sense, energy body of astral- emotional and spiritual, Planet of Venus.

Qualities of compassion, gentleness, lightness. Related to the sense of touch and relationship. Giving and receiving Divine Love transcends the ego.

Balanced energy is compassion, can see good in everyone, has a desire to nurture others and is friendly and outgoing.

Unbalanced feels sorry for oneself, paranoid, indecisive, afraid of letting go, being free, getting hurt, being abandoned or demanding, overly critical, tense between the shoulder blades, possessive, moody, melodramatic, attitude of a martyr.

Fifth Chakra located at the base of the neck, is the colour of blue and turquoise.

Note of G, Element of Either, gland of thyroid, sense of hearing, Energy body = spiritual body, and Planets of Mercury and Neptune.

Relates to communication and self-expression vocation and quality of receptivity.

Balanced means the ability to speak ones own truth, self-expression in society, profession. Receptivity and the ability to take responsibility for one's own needs.

Unbalanced means suppressing self, introvert, timid, scared, sullen, inability to articulate or express oneself emotionally, fear of failure **or** arrogant, self righteous, talk too much, dogmatic.

Sixth Chakra is located in the third eye, brow area and is the colour of indigo. Note of A., Element of Mind, glands of Pineal, pituitary, Energy bodies of spiritual and soul bodies ruled by the Planet Jupiter.

Relates to the positive thinking, insight, and clairvoyance. Ability to experience telepathy, astral travels and past lives. Connected to the ability to visualise and perceive mental concepts, imagination.

Balanced means mastering the power of positive thought.

Unbalanced means confused mental concepts, images of reality are not true and negative, non-assertive, afraid of success and has ability to generate strong negative ideas, **or** egotistical pride, manipulative, religiously dogmatic.

Seventh Chakra is located on top of the head and is a violet or white colour and if very spiritual the person color is gold and magenta.

Note of B., Element cosmic energy and thought, Glands of pituitary, pineal, Energy body Soul - body, Planet of Uranus.

Relates to the experience of oneness of God, All that is, experience beyond duality, The connection between the personal self and the universe Center of self- realisation, Relationship with father and the I AM.

Balanced means open to the divine, sense of alignment with higher forces, integration of whole being, physical, emotional, mental and spiritual.

Unbalanced no spark or joy, cannot make decisions, no conscious connection to one's own spirituality or constant sense of frustration, unrealised power, depressed, migraine headaches, destructive.

I do not believe in reinventing the wheel and when I see a good product I will mention it, so if you would like a good colour plate and explanation of the 7 Chakras similar to those mentioned, write to Crystal Reflections PO Box 1853 Auckland New Zealand.

CRYSTAL and GEMSTONE HEALING

There seems to be a lot of mystical things said about crystal and gemstone healing, and long ago I learnt what to do and how to place the crystals on the body for maximum benefit. Some really good results were achieved using the vibration of the crystal to enhance a lost or unbalanced energy in the intricate patterning or webbing in the body and aura.

To me crystals are like little batteries that can be programmed negatively or positively and really enhance your own energy when you are holding them.

It is very important to cleanse them of all energy after you purchase them as they will pick up and transmit stressful, negative or positive energies from the place you have purchased them.
It is also important to cleanse them every six months even if they are just lying around the house.
I find that putting your crystals or gemstones in salt water for 24 hours grounds the negative energies. After washing the salt off them with filtered water, bury them in the soft dirt for 24 hours and then leave them in the moonlight overnight and the indirect sunlight the following day for a short time to restore all the elemental energies. Then be quiet, hold the crystal and imagine a stairwell going down into the crystal. Travel in the crystal and ask to talk to the crystal guardian and after greeting it with respect tell it what you want it to do for you and what symbols you will use to instruct it to help you.

For example, if you want it to shield you from negative energies then you might use a symbol of a sword. For healing to take place maybe a healing hand or a symbol of God's healing praying hands. To help you get an answer for your direction maybe a book of wisdom. By projecting this symbol through the crystal you may be pleasantly surprised what help you can get.
Never underestimate the power of crystals.

One of the best crystal healings I ever had was with an intuitive lady who is very modest in her work. She laid out lots of crystals and gemstones around me and placed them according to the vibration of the Chakras on the body. Talk about an out of body experience. WOW! Helen Burne lives in Phoenix Arizona USA and can be contacted through the writer as she really enjoys her privacy.

There are many good books on Crystal Healing. Focus on Crystals by Edmund Harold is one that will take the mystique out of it all.
The adjoining photo was taken in sunlight by Gene Falk of Sedona Arizona with a special lens and shows the kinetic energy coming out of the body of the crystal.

Gene also has a magnificent video which when viewed will put even the most stressed person into a rested state of Alpha and has been used in hospital and medical waiting rooms with great success.

I played one of the videos at a New Age party on the request of the hostess. The party was pretty well tanked up and by the time the tape finished everyone was falling asleep. I did warn the hostess.

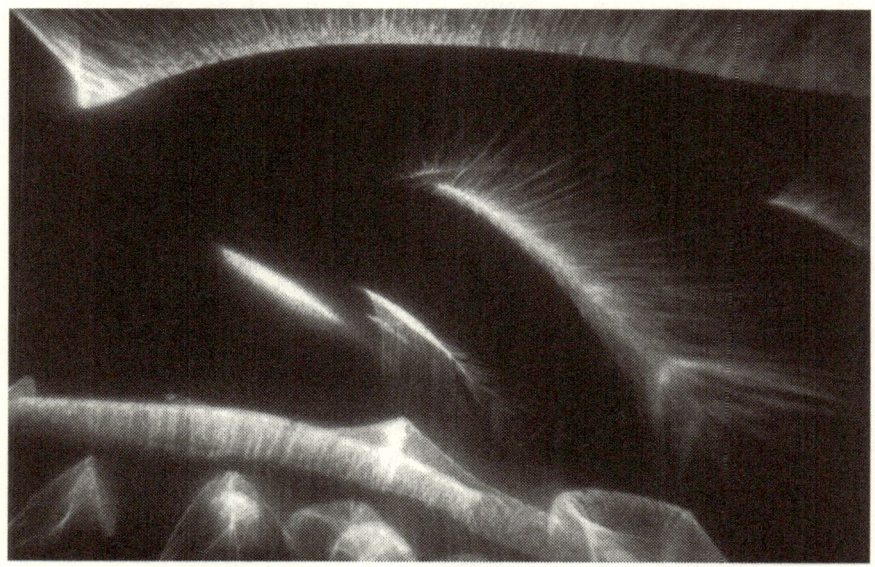

Kinetic energy coming from a crystal outside in the sunlight, photograph by Mr Gene Falk.

The Ancients have used gemstones for centuries. In ancient times in China you would go to a dowser who would dowse for the type of mineral you needed. He would proceed to grind the mineral/ gemstone, add it to water for the patient to drink and the patient would be cured, some times. Energy and chemical healing? I would not recommend this, as some minerals are toxic to the body.

Gemstones

Gemstones were worn as power stones to increase the power vibrations by royalty and nobility, while church priests in different religions and even the Popes are adorned. Still today gemstones adorn their crowns, swords, clothing and such. They are not always used as ornaments and glitter as the next section will show you.

If you wish to find out which gemstones empower you purchase a pendulum and dowse to see which gemstones empower your energies then carry them with you or place on the hurting area of your body. There are now special beds and mattresses made up with gemstones layered into them that are great to experience and it is surprising how sometimes pain energy moves while on the bed.

Ancient Healing Stones

AMAZONITE (Green/Blue) - Encourages faith and hope. Regulates thinking faculties.

AMBER (Gold) - Lifts the spirits, neutralize infections, respiratory diseases.

AMETHYST (Purple) - Headaches, alcoholism, overindulgence, meditation, spiritual wisdom negative energies.

ANGEL SKIN CORAL (Coral) - Arthritis, throat and voice, promotes a sense of well-being.

AQUAMARINE (Aqua to Light Blue) - Calming of nerves, aids in marine travel, eyesight, reduces fluid retention.

AZURITE and MALACHITE (Blue and Green) - Cancer prevention, develops psychic abilities, powerful healing stone, mental control and balance, optic nerve, success in business, aids fertility, arthritis.

BANDED AGATE (Brown-Orange) - Strength and courage.

BLACK CORAL (Black) - Balances physical energy, relaxing tension, respiratory infection.

BLACK JADE (Black) - Dispels negativity, wisdom, long life, peaceful death.

BLOODSTONE (Dark Green/Red) - High blood pressure, physical trauma, blood circulation, bloodshot eyes, stimulates flow of energy.

BLUE LACE AGATE (Light Blue) - Happiness, emotional tranquillity, balances body fluids, temper.

BLUE QUARTZ (Blue) - Jealousy, patience.

BLUE SAPPHIRE (Blue) - Wisdom, spiritual enlightenment, mental clarity, protection, relieves mental depression, peace and happiness, motivation to achieve goals.

BROWN JASPER (Brown) - Gives emotional security, aids female hormonal functions, safety in operation of machinery.

CARNELIAN (Orange-Red) - Energy, feeling of well-being, protection, liver, gallbladder, pancreas.

CHRYSOPRASE (Green) - Sedative, tranquilliser, inferiority complexes, all mental problems.

CITRINE (Yellow) - Colon, gall bladder, liver, digestive tract.

DENDRITE AGATE (Gray/Brown) - Traveller's stone, security and endurance, low blood sugar, car travel.

EMERALD (Green) - Creativity, memory, problem solving, neurological diseases, perception.

EYE AGATE (Black Spots) - Counteracts negative thinking, protects from bodily harm.

FOSSIL (Brown Shell) - Increases domestic efficiency, increases potassium, magnesium, calcium.

GARNET (Purple) - Bloodstream, arthritis, circulation, hormones, popularity, thyroid.

GREEN JADE (Green) - Stomach disorders, eases eyestrain, liver, good luck, wisdom and practicality.

GREEN JASPER (Green) - Constipation, colon, intestinal tract.

GREEN MOSS AGATE (Green) - Cleans blood, balance, balances discordant emotional energies.

GREEN QUARTZ (Green) - Feet, leg problems, joints, digits (fingers and toes).

GREEN TOURMALINE (Green) - Attracts success and wealth, prevents lymphatic diseases, battles anaemia.

INDIA AGATE (Gray) - Physical strength.

IVORY (Cream) - Protects from physical injury, klutziness.

JASPER (Green or Red) - Healing of gastric system, safety in operation of machinery.

JET (Black) - Effective against evil thoughts and deep depression, protection stone.

LAPIS LAZULI (Blue) - Intelligence, creativity, ESP powers, wisdom, fidelity, truthfulness.

SHELLS (Many Colors) - Increases potassium, magnesium, calcium, household efficiency.

SMOKY QUARTZ (Brown) - Calms nerves, sedative, relaxant, hypnosis.

SODALITE (Blue) - Thyroid, diabetes, courage, endurance, dispels guilt and fears.

SPECKLED AGATE (Speckled Gray/Brown) - Air travel.

PECTROLITE (Gray) - Helps bad backs, inspiration, spleen, sexual deficiencies, and pituitary gland.

TIGER-EYE (Brown) Clear THINKING memory, bloodstream, headaches and nervous spasms, psychic protector.

TOPAZ CRYSTAL (Light Brown) - Fights kidney and bladder ailments, lung disorders, asthma, eyes.

TOURMALINE - WATERMELON (Multicolored) - Cancer prevention, good for success and management.

TREE AGATE (White and Green) - Relieves tension, reduces fever and toxins, physical and emotional balance.

TURQUOISE (Turquoise) - Protect ion stone, inner joy and peace, aids mental relaxation, calms emotions.

WHITE JADE (White) - Good luck stone, eyes, nervous system, dispels negativity.

YELLOW JASPER (Yellow/Gold) - Constipation, colon, intestinal tract.

Maybe now you know why you have been attracted to a certain crystal or gemstone to provide energy you need.

Do not under any circumstance grind up any of these stones and take them internally. This was an ancient art that has been lost to us when books were destroyed by those fearful of things they did not understand and in the interests of self preservation destroyed most of the knowledge.

Pendulum Instructions

If you cannot afford to purchase some of the fine-tuned solid brass - precision pendulums then what I suggest is this. My mother used a needle and thread to find out the sex of a child before it was born this way so it doesn't have to be expensive to work.
Find a clear crystal that has a point on one end and tie it to some string or double strength cotton so the point is pointing down and reasonably balanced when lifted up. Make sure the crystal has been blessed or cleansed first or bless it yourself in the name of whomever you believe in. Hold it in the palm of your hand and give it your love and vibration before using. Say a prayer over it or energise it with your own loving energy if you wish.
Hold the pendulum between thumb and forefinger with your elbow on the table to brace it to steady it and ground yourself. Relax and think of nothing except that you only want the truth and nothing but the truth. No ego strokers here.

Before asking questions you need to establish the yes /no answers and this can be done in the early stages by putting a cross on a piece of paper like north, south, east, west lines as below.

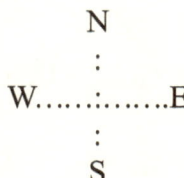

```
        N
        ┊
W...........┊.......E
        ┊
        S
```

Then swinging gently along the north south line state out loud as though you are talking to a trusted buddy "this for a yes."

Along the east west line "this for a no."

In a anticlockwise direction circle "this if you do not understand the question, a no or when clearing negative energy from the body."

In a clockwise direction circle, "This if you are healing in a positive balancing mode or a yes."

Then practice formulating questions that you know the answers to and are obvious, to get familiar with the process. It does take time but can be a really helpful aid as one can develop a direct link to one's own subconscious mind which knows all about you.

All questions however must be phrased so they can be answered with a yes or no answer and if you are not sure then ask if such and such answer is the truth.

There are many classes on this field and there are many professional dowsers who have found water by using this method and also rods for divining. Practice and a clear mind detached from the out come brings accuracy and suggest while learning to do this do it away from others as they may try to alter your answers with their mind power in an effort to manipulate. Spiritual Response Therapy and workshops with Robert Detzler for advanced pendulum work is organized at Spiritual Response Center 727 245 Th Place NE, Redmond WA 98053 or 206-868-3643

SE-5 INFORMATION

The following information is about an instrument I have used for approximately ten years and the health of myself and my family has improved beyond that I had even envisioned. My friends have begun to say each time they see me that I am looking younger and more vital every year and I do attribute a lot of this to the SE-5 Intrinsic Data Field Analyzer which still classed as a research instrument. The SE-5 is an incredible instrument for analysis and balancing of the subtle energies and I firmly believe that every household should own one.

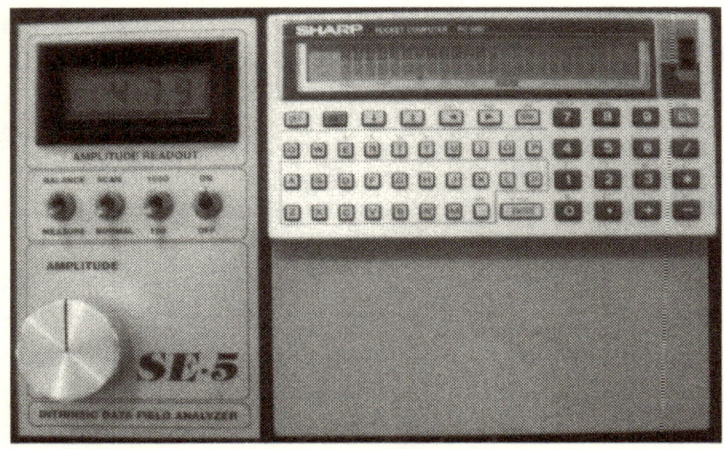

Following the information about the SE-5, I have included some of the incredible things that others and I have experienced from the use of the SE-5. UNBELIEVABLE to say the least.

CONCEPTS AND PRINCIPLES IN IDF RESEARCH

EVERYTHING IN THE UNIVERSE IS ENERGY IN ITS MOST FUNDAMENTAL FORM AND ALL FORMS OF ENERGY ARE GOVERENED BY INTRINSIC DATA FIELDS (IDF's). Energy exists everywhere as potential and in motion creates fields allowing energy to be transmitted, absorbed and conducted.

Energy exists in spirit as consciousness, in mind as thoughts, in emotion as feelings, in electricity, in magnetism and gravitation as force fields, in the physical as molecular mass and in an energy exchange as communication. Light, sound, heat, magnetism, color, electricity, are all just different forms of the same source....energy. They differ only in frequency of vibration and the medium of conduction.

Like a tuning fork energy vibrates, oscillates and resonates at specific frequencies. At one or more frequencies a thought is formed, at another an emotion felt, at another an object is created, at still another an environment is formed from complex wave patterns of subtle information.

The air we breathe, the food we eat, the people we know, our thoughts, feelings and our body as well as the environment in which we live is fundamentally concentrated energy fields existing at different frequencies.

Like all objects, the body radiates and absorbs frequency waves of energy. Each of our senses: seeing, hearing, tasting, smelling and touching, work through energies at specific frequency bands along the electromagnetic spectrum. (The electromagnetic spectrum is a chart which illustrates man's and nature's activity in the use of electromagnetic energy in terms of a common denominator: frequency. The spectrum is a graduated table of all known frequencies or rates of vibration.)

We tend only to believe that which we can sense, but our five senses perceive only a limited frequency band of the spectrum. We are actually unaware of most of the energies that exist. We cannot see the emanations of police radar, the energy halos around TV transmitters or VHF radio antenna, or X-rays. Yet each of these devices produces electromagnetic energies. There is a greater reality than what appears to be. One needs only consider that until electricity was discovered and applied it was thought not to exist, but it had always been there, ready to be used. Our bodies may appear to be solid, but if we magnify the cells, molecules, and atoms of which we are composed we would see that at the most basic level we are made up of subtle information fields containing little if any matter. We are not just physical and chemical structures, but beings composed of energy.

Just what is a field? A magnet that attracts iron may be placed under a sheet of cardboard. Iron particles sprinkled on the cardboard will align themselves in patterns around the magnet. Scientists call these patterns "lines of magnetic force." A collection of these lines around a magnet, in three dimensions, is called a magnetic field.

A radio broadcasting station radiates an electromagnetic field from its tower. This field of energy may be mapped out or measured with electric field strength meters.

The gravitational field surrounding the earth may be mapped by measuring the earth's attraction for a small mass. Plotting such measurements describes a gravitational field.

All animate and inanimate objects such as minerals, chemicals and living things are surrounded with Intrinsic Data Fields. These are informational fields that structure energy into form or patterns. These fields relate to the objects or energies inside their fields.

Each year more scientific evidence accumulates bringing us closer to the realization that our health and well-being may be more related to the function of IDFs operating in and around our body.

With the advent of quantum mechanics a new perspective of life is emerging as research delves into the nature of the creative forces which produce matter. Fifteen years ago most of the electromagnetic spectrum was empty. Today, with more sophisticated measurement instrumentation, it is practically full. Science is finding that it is not the strong high voltage high intensity energies which cause the most change, but the lower more subtle energies which are closer or more attuned to cellular communications in the body. Instruments such as the SQUID at M.I.T., Kirlian photographs, tensiometers, and nuclear magnetic resonators have been used to detect extremely subtle information fields emanating from all objects.

These latest discoveries show how subtle information forces in nature can penetrate everything, cause instantaneous reaction at incredible distances, do not behave according to known formulas, cannot be measured by conventional electronic test equipment, and represent a completely new spectrum of energy.

The references to this spectrum have been given many names such as: the second force of gravity, eloptics, dowsing, radionics, radiesthesia, psionics, scalar waves, bioplasm, and the ethers, LFields, prana, Kirlian effect, chi, auras, orgone, the pre-physical state, the body electric, Intrinsic Data Fields (IDFs) or biofield. Regardless of the name, these subtle energies or biofields are said to contain the intelligence or information which provides the pattern (or energy matrix) for the organization of matter. We call these informational patterns IDFs (Intrinsic Data Fields). In many instances these phenomena can explain things that cannot be explained by orthodox science.

Just as an architect prepares a blueprint for a structure to be built, similarly subtle information fields contain information, i.e. IDFs, (similar to a microfilm) is a plan for how energy will be organized and structured into matter.

BIOFIELDS

The biofield has been described as a complex multi-structured system with the physical body representing the lowest aspect in the levels of control. Our physical body is a dense mirror reflection of the biofield.

The biofield serves as a communications device, a receiving and transmission system for converting coded information signals of energy into thought, emotion and behavior patterns as well as the life forming and healing powers of the physical body. The biofield also governs ionization or processing of nutrients into physical energy where opposite polarities attract and is a transducer of subtle cosmic and nuclear high frequency energies where opposite polarities repel and like attracts like.

The concept of everything being an information field or biofield now occupies the most advanced thinking in our scientific community. As scientists unveil the layers of energy of the human being, we are beginning to reformulate the definition of ourselves as energy receivers and transmitters.

This new definition includes the existence of other bodies or dimensions besides the physical. The biofield appears to contain:
1. A spiritual body manifesting as awareness, consciousness, intent or will.

2. A mental body composed of attitudes, beliefs, ideas, abstract and concrete thoughts and a recording of all our experiences.

3. An emotional body composed of feelings, sensation and desires.

4. An etheric body or an energetic pattern of the physical which contains the pattern template for the structure and function of the physical body and the IDF circuits as the meridians and energy centers such as the charkas.

5. A physical body (the result of all the bodies) composed of chemicals and tissue.

6. A multi-dimensional system of energy communication and transmission between the various bodies called chakras or energy centers corresponding to the endocrine glands and neural plexus. Every physical part, function and imbalance has its counterpart which is built from etheric, emotional and mental energies. The concept of these subtle bodies may seem to be metaphysical but only because most of our awareness in western cultures is focused on the physical.

All of these bodies can be seen as vibrations or auras existing at different energies. Thought forms, habits, beliefs, values, emotional qualities are all frequency patterns of energy. We tune into our mind energy by thinking, our emotional energy by feeling and physical energy through the sensory and motor responses of the nervous system.

The biofield model is being conceptualized as an informational field expressing itself as individual and collective mind existing in a state of subtle electromagnetic and gravitational wave patterns.

Scientists are now advancing the proposal that these subatomic subtle electromagnetic and gravitational-like fields form a holographic representation which may not only serve as the control mechanism for matter, but may very well be how consciousness or mind expresses itself into matter.

This energy information may be how our thoughts, emotions and bodies are created. Subatomic particle waves manifesting as light and sound are being considered the connecting link between consciousness, energy and matter.

Light and sound provide a means for continuity of process between matter and mind. The cause of all things may be in the subatomic field in which the mind, through vibrations of light and sound, plays a creative role, much like a movie (mind) projects its images of light and sound onto the screen (called matter). Matter is more accurately perceived as frozen light and sound.

The hologram is a three dimensional image picture taken with laser light. You can cut the film over and over and still be able to see the entire image in the hologram energy pattern. Brain researchers offer the hologram as the best explanation of how we work. Every cell contains representational information of the whole, e.g. the macrocosm is contained in the microcosm.

The biofield is a vibrational force which surrounds and inter-penetrates all matter. It appears to organize free energy at specific frequencies which in turn manifest and give shape and dimension to physical form. Simple energies form a basic yet different element, each of which are defined in Chemistry's Periodic Table of The Elements. Matter is simply an organized pattern of vibrations. ..trapped energy as it were.

The biofield patterns of energy are first evident as subtle electromagnetic fields at the subatomic level. As the field density increases, or crystallizes, an electrical potential or charge is created at a specific level. The electrical charges manifest as the various elements and provide the chemical bonding for the states of matter such as gases, liquids and solids. The character of energy is first electromagnetic before it becomes molecular. As such the biofield also appears to govern the regulation of chemical processes from the simple cell up through the human being.

As a result of this flow of energy from the most subtle to the densest, disorders and degeneration in matter appear to result initially from imbalances in the subtle energies or biofields. Conversely balanced biofields appear to supply energy to maintain a healthy state of matter.

INSTRUMENTATION

With recent advances in physics and computer technology researchers are now able to measure and influence the subtle energies surrounding the body and objects in the environment. Instruments have been developed to expand and amplify our senses to form a communication link with the subtle biofield energies.

Instruments can now detect the informational contents of the biofield to locate imbalances or interferences in the flow of energy and to change or modify the energetic qualities of life.

At the forefront in IDF research instrumentation is the SE-S plus Intrinsic Data Field Analyzer developed by physicist Willard Frank. This device combines the best features of previous instrumentation, is computerized for rapid processing of information and is compatible with most personal computers for increased memory capability.

The SE-S plus INTRINSIC DATA FIELD ANALYZER, popularly known as the SE-S, is a solid state electronic instrument designed to detect, quantify and transmit a full spectrum of IDF signals to restore normal wave form patterns or functions of the biofield.

Designed as a Spectrometer to analyze the energies emitted by mineral samples, the SE-S's use as an experimental research device has increased dramatically with the discovery of subtle information fields surrounding living systems.

The SE-S plus has as its mechanism of operation the fundamental principles of energy fields.

More specifically stated, the instrument 1) measures IDF radiation of an object and 2) transmits IDF wave patterns to the object.

The SE-S plus, therefore, does not operate directly on the physical level but functions as a receiver, transmitter and modulator of wave form information found in the subatomic or subtle magnetic and gravitational energy fields which precede the manifestation of matter in its elemental and molecular form.

All matter, through radiation, emits energy and absorbs energy at predictable levels. The SE-S plus as a research device can be used to analyze and communicate with the subtle informational content of matter. The instrument assists the operator in establishing, through electronic means, a conscious link with subtle body/mind energies.

The laws and principles of energy instrumentation are therefore not that of Newtonian physics but are grounded in concepts of advanced Quantum mechanics, resonance, harmony, reinforcement, interference, balance and imbalance. Any organism is strengthened and weakened based on its relationship to these terms.

IDF research with the SE-S plus is thus an attempt to analyze energy fields and IDFs to:
1. Determine resonance or dissonance (imbalances) at specific levels.
2. Neutralize imbalance and support weak fields.
3. Balance the levels of natural energies. This is achieved by tuning into a specific energy level to communicate like a two way radio.

A biofield instrument assists in measuring IDFs which contain information about the contents of that field. Balancing experiments send corrective information back to the energy field under study, suggesting that a subtle information balancing action take place.

Just how these IDFs interface or represent, like a blueprint, the structure and function of matter and how the instrumentation can be used to analyze and influence these IDFs is now discussed.

MASS. MOLECULES AND FORM: THE PHYSICAL STATE

Scientifically we know that all substance has its form by virtue of its molecular arrangement. Investigation has demonstrated that the molecule is the basic mass-form upon which all substance having shape is built. To be sure, scientists have electrically broken down the molecule into the smaller particles of chemical elements, ions and atoms, but these are not mass- forms. Hence the molecule is the accepted mass-structure unit for matter.

Electrophysiological studies have established conclusively that the electrical potentials found in the human body are directly related to electrical patterns; this pattern dictates the nature of the organism. The pattern is a dynamic process, not static, which allows the organism to grow, mature, regenerate and evolve.

The organism builds new cells but they are always organized according to the original electrical pattern, e.g., an acorn becomes an oak tree not a cabbage. The patterning is determined in the subatomic field of frequency vibration which play themselves out on the pre-physical level in the DNA of the cell. The pattern is recreated in the newly emerging cells.

Mention should here be made of how Yale University research workers Burr and Northrop succeeded in establishing conclusive evidence - after probing with a sensitive voltmeter the subtle electrical variations which accompany all process of growth - that the electrical potential found in the human body is directly related to an electrical pattern.

The Burr and Northrop studies established conclusively that the electrical potential found in the human body is directly related to an electrical pattern; this pattern dictates the nature of the organism, but it is not an inflexible form; rather it is a patterning principle in the sense that it evolves and changes. As the patterning evolves, so the organism evolves, assumes form, grows, matures, remains constant; then the organism builds new cells, but always organizes them after the original design. The organism is recreated, but always with the pattern dictated. The patterning here is a dynamic process, not a static entity. The patterning has an implicit form that it communicates to the organism. The patterning is determined in the subatomic field and given the same environment, it evolves with fidelity; electrical vibration here is a force. This force works to incarnate the patterning in the emerging cellular entity: to form the lion, the rose, the man, the diamond, the drop of oil, illness, health. It is the pulsating rhythm of form and pattern that is termed life. It is potential, patterning, and form that reflect the three principles of structural integrity, organism- rejuvenation and regeneration.

The shape or form of a substance is directly dependent upon the arrangement and variation of the millions of molecules which compose it. Thus the substance of wood differs from that of cloth; earth from water; flesh from metal; one wood from another; one metal from another; one tissue from another. Every recognizable form assumes that form because of the molecules of which it is composed. It has a definite arrangement peculiar to itself, and differing from all others.

For instance, the chemical molecules in the air become a form of substance which we recognize as rain; with a different molecular arrangement of those same chemicals we have, instead, snow; still another, and we have sleet; another and we have hail; yet another and we have steam or mist. But the chemical content has remained identical throughout. Thus, when we note differences in mass substances we are virtually recognizing them by their variations in molecular arrangement. When we look into a microscope and say, "This is kidney tissue, this is liver" etc., we are identifying them not only by their form and their structural tissue but also by their molecular variations.

In addition, we know that these molecules are in constant motion, adhering together by force fields which animate the substance and which, when no longer present, allows it to disintegrate through a molecular separation and alteration in the mass-form. Some call this death, or say the mind or soul has moved on. Science defines energy as motion, and energy in the form of the motion of molecules and their arrangement is different as the form varies. For instance, the energy emanating from the activity of liver tissue would be different from that of the kidney, thyroid, stomach, pancreas, pituitary, or any other tissue of the body. When we recognize one form as varying from others we are likewise recognizing it by its difference in energy production.

Life is a manifestation of a ceaseless exchange between various degrees of matter. The character of the energy implanted in the body during that activity is, above all, electronic energy before it is ionic and before it becomes molecular, for it proceeds from the sphere of vibration. We only perceive the secondary physical effects, those which manifest on the plane of matter and which are recognized as molecular activity.

The purely physical approach is the basis of biochemistry. The emphasis is on molecular activity as though it were the only reality. Our orthodox scientists either forget or are unaware that molecular activity relates only to a final group and not to the fundamental impulses which cause or stimulate these molecules into activity.

INTRISIC DATA FIELDS: THE PRE-PHYSICAL STATE

Since science has demonstrated that a substance composed of moving parts will vibrate in accordance with the motion of those parts, just as an automobile vibrates according to the slowness or rapidity of motion of the parts comprising the engine, then these various substance forms, these tissues, will have a subtle vibration, pattern or rate, directly proportional to the molecular activity composing them, just as distinctive to those tissue forms as the arrangement of their molecules or the energy they produced. Everything exists in its natural state as long as the normal vibrational pattern exists. (It may be interesting to note that even machines have their own energy fields which can be detected and altered.)

Atoms act like little radio transmitters broadcasting waves. Humans, as well as all kinds of supposedly inert matter, constantly emit rays. Every metal and every person sends out waves of different lengths. Personal wave lengths are as individual as fingerprints.

Thus, under the laws of vibration each individual has distinctive rates of vibration or resonance harmonics. Each person and each individual part of our body produces different patterns of vibrational tones and energies. Each of us, in effect, are like tuning forks trying to maintain our proper note. Each organ, gland and tissue has its own vibration rate as well. All cells are the same until differentiation or specialization occurs as a result of a group harmonic. There is a subtle information principle of formative subtle energies guarding the integration of matter and controlling the structural replication and differentiation of all organisms.

If you strike a note on a piano you get a simple vibration. Another note with the necessary harmonic together will form a chord. There are untold numbers of vibrations and each has a definite wave length and is analogous to a single note on the piano. All frequencies have their own relationship and harmonic.

Hence, the energy radiating from every tissue does so in harmonics resonating or vibrational wavelengths peculiar to that organ or tissue and in proportion to the vibration3 of the tissue as represented by the molecular activity within it. In the same way one radio wave will resonate with another radio wave. We can regard resonance and harmonics as an affinity or the valency, the power of one element to combine with another such as found in chemical elements. Applying this to the subtle energies, the imbalances are only altered energies to the normal harmonic or resonance. Our bodies are virtually a composite of many vibrations constantly creating energy, constantly sending out and taking in energy according to each biofield pattern or blueprint of activity.

BIOFIELD ANALYSIS

Just as a commercial radio "tunes in" on wavelengths of sound or energy sent out from a commercial broadcasting station, so do IDF instruments such as the SE-S calibrate or "tune in" on energies sent out from our tissue "broadcasting" stations. The SE-5 is a quantum mechanical tuning fork acts as a receiving set for the reception of the various energies.

A medical drug works because the radiations which it emits have the right harmonic relationship with those of the disease and the part of the body being affected. A part of the wave form being emitted by the drug forms a discord with the radiations of the disease.

The SE-S is so constructed that operators report being able selectively to "tune in" to the various IDFs of the organs, glands and tissues of the body and receive the specific wavelengths of information being emitted. Then, by precise tuning, the degree of variation in that wavelength reception from the normal point can be determined, and the degree of variation in the energy production and activity can be interpreted.

Invading organisms, abnormal tissue formations and emotional and mental states have their own molecular arrangements, electrical charges and IDF vibrational patterns. The IDF presence may be detected by tuning in to their particular levels. Hence, the researchers report using the SE-S to conduct differential analyses as well as charting of IDF levels associated with organs, glands, tissues, systems, feelings, thoughts and environmental patterns.

Other vibration wavelengths may also be detected when the SE-S's computer is set for the reception of a subtle information pattern from a particular part of the body for a specific imbalance. If this imbalance is present, it is broadcasting incessantly and it is said that when we "tune in" for that energy we receive its "broadcast."

If it is not present, even though we have analyzed for this energy, we receive no broadcast since it has been "assigned" to one molecular arrangement alone. Complete analyses of any subject matter may be done in this manner. Each tissue has its own mass-form and therefore its own IDF pattern which researchers report can be measured. The same principles may apply to any state of energy such as thoughts, emotions, environments, relationships between people, and even events and situations all have their unique characteristic energy signature.

To conduct an analysis, a sample of the subject's hair, saliva or photograph, optimally a Polaroid photograph is placed inside the specimen tray of the instrument. This sample appears to serve as a target for locating the actual bio field in time/space. The research operator manipulates the various keys of the computer and, moving the fingers over the detector plate on the instrument, selectively tunes in to these vibrations. The plate is used because, to date, the human nervous system provides the best antenna for detecting subtle energies. Researchers state this mechanism is made possible by the fact that when the lower vibratory wavelengths of energy, such as are found in imbalances or lowered-functioning parts (which energy is negative to the total body energy) meets the positive energy or flow of subatomic particles from the operator's hand, a direct short, or "stick," is noted on the detector plate. Thus, by introducing varying resistances with different key changes, the operator may shift from one wavelength reception to another, from one subtle information organ, gland or tissue to another, and determines the deviation in relation to normal. Normal being 0 for negative subtle energies and the subject's vitality or 100 measure being normal for positive energies.

For analysis the instrument has several automatic subject area programs and any number of word frequency rates can be entered manually. The SE-S was designed to first measure energies that may be out of resonance with the natural occurring patterns. This may be due to some obstructed energy channel of the body. When such obstruction occurs, the energy may no longer vibrate to the rate of the total body energy, but sets up a lower vibration of its own causing interferences and imbalances. The SE-S operator may then proceed to detect negative vibrational energies which should not be present in the biofield.

Researchers report that these energy imbalances and blockages occurring in the field are usually due to trauma, stress, abuses, deficiencies, outside pathogens or auto-intoxication and immune dysfunction. The imbalances create subtle information resistance of excessive amplitude at specific wavelengths in the normal vibration of the biofield. The imbalances may manifest themselves in many signs and signals as: mental and emotional disorders, obstruction in meridians, discomfort, pain and distress, etc. Most disturbances are detectable in the pre-physical state of matter long before they manifest physically.

Disease and disorder may also be caused by interferences in the natural harmonics or vibrational patterns. The primary objective may be the removal of these interferences and to correct the harmonic balance.

With the SE-S plus, researchers relate that it is possible to have an accurate and detailed picture of IDF structure and function. Analysis by "guess" can be substantially eliminated which is a definite aid to every researcher regardless of profession.

BIOFIELD BALANCING

Now that we have made an analysis with this instrument, what, then, may we do with this information? Researchers first put the SE-S plus into its balancing mode. The keyboard and computer screen on the instrument assume the role of control for the energies desired. The amplitude knob is designed to either increase or lower the amplitude of the IDF. The SE-S plus has been said to perform the IDF balancing just as the vibration of a tuning fork or piano string is "stepped up" or "retarded," as the case may be, to harmonize with the wavelength of that energy being sent against it in the tuning process.

The energy of a wave form is maximized when wavelengths are in resonance or vibrating at similar levels. The further the deviation from the natural resonance the greater the resistance and loss of productive energy available to that object. The SE-S plus has been compared to a resonator or oscillator designed to reestablish the natural frequency resonance of an object. In this process the SE-S plus seems to use the energy of the research subjects as a carrier wave to both receive and transmit frequency information.

The accuracy in analysis is very important as the researcher conducts balancing experiments. Some say, if an arbitrary stimulation is selected, only a temporary or marginal effect is produced. Others say if the exact energy needed is introduced, the response is more vigorous, and resonance is amplified many fold as a result of the exactness of synchronism of the resonance. Still other researchers say as the IDF vibration of a tissue is altered, so, indirectly, may electrical potentials and eventually its molecular activity and function change. But just how is this accounted for from a physiological perspective.

Resonance explains many things which have puzzled doctors and biologists. How is it that certain constituents of the blood such as hormones and enzymes, though minute in size, exert such a powerful influence and moreover one that is localized. It may be that these substances are exceedingly subtle yet strong centers of radiation and that they act only on cells of the body whose radiations are in resonance with theirs.

As stated previously, research in quantum physics has demonstrated that the subtle energies are, by nature, sound and light waves. This invisible energy may be received in its own wavelengths in the instrument and any deviation from the normal can be noted and measured.

This energy, which activates our tissues, is said to be in the nature of light. A common experiment of the biology laboratory is that of sending a beam of light against a one-celled organism and noting the effect of that beam in intensifying the activity within the nucleus of the cell until cleavage of cell nucleus finally takes place. Experiments currently under way at one university are using laser as a carrier wave of subtle information to duplicate effects of medicinal substances in a target specimen.

The application of these scientific facts may answer the question as to what occurs with use of the SE-S plus. We have subtle energy of scalar waves -- an "energy beam," if you please -- being sent into the sample at the wavelength energies of that sample itself

The new wavelengths of substance particles are said to interact with the process of metabolism and cell division. In one year every cell dies and is regenerated. If you read this paper a year from now you are a completely new you. Since this process is constantly going on in the body, the new cells will come in at the higher rate of vibration and the imbalanced cells will automatically fall away. A normalizing effect may occur as long as the correct pattern of the biofield is maintained. The immune system may simply be this higher rate of vibration. As like poles repel and unlike poles attract, cell division obviously takes place when the invisible vibrations, positive in their polarity, strike the positively charged nucleus of the cell. Abnormal interfering vibrations can no more continue to exist in normally vibrating tissue than light and darkness can exist in the same spot.

BIOFIELD ANALYSIS AND BALANCING

Here one point must be made clear. In analysis we wish to receive the IDF emanating or radiating from the negative energy formation itself, and we deal with that alone. In balancing, however, the negative energy is not sent back into the sample in its own vibration. The computer settings neutralize the transmission of the negative energy and reduce it. The computer screen information and transmission may control both negative IDF conditions and locations into which neutralizing energy is sent.

For instance, in analysis some investigators report a negative IDF imbalance or problems (not the physical condition itself) in the lung and utilize that same keyboard or computer screen setting for balancing. We are following a pattern of localizing the IDF imbalance in the lung by tuning into that lung, and by further analysis specifying the IDF condition of the lung. Both location and condition are identified for reception of the energy wavelengths which will lead to balancing and or neutralization.

The operator is not eliminating the unbalanced tissue by concentration of its own rate, but is said to normalize the IDF vibratory process in that particular area. Through this process, the normal may exclude the abnormal of its own accord, and a healthy state will be created. Any long-term imbalances may require work on the pre-physical state of matter as well as the physical in order to provide long-term changes.

In the same way that researchers tune in on the various IDF functions and imbalances, they report being able to tune in on reagents or remedies for the elimination of those vibrations. Homeopathic physicians, particularly, have reported the SE-S plus instrument invaluable because of its accuracy and exactness in researching homeopathic remedies and potency needed for the dissipation of energy imbalances.

It cannot be too greatly stressed that the individual's own subtle information body is the only force or current used by the SE-S plus in analysis, reagent selection or balancing. There are no physical energies connected in any way with the instrument. Were this the case the individuals' own rate of vibration or the flow of their own energy would not control the SE-S plus' output. Suppose we made a mistake in analysis. In that event we may not be directing the IDF properly into the part desired. Even if there was a mistake, subtle energies sent into that area would be reflected if not needed. This may not do any good if there were no imbalances but it also can do no harm. We thus find reports that the operating principles of the SE-S plus are supportive to one's own biofield because it is working with or controlled by the subtle information frequency patterns of the research subject.

Analysis and balancing by means of this instrument is an entirely informational process. Investigators report that it communicates normalizing energy to any system. These energies may gradually take the place of imbalanced (subtle) formations caused by wrong thinking, emotional stress or continuous physical abuse and injuries.

The SE-S plus it is said measures pre-physical energy beneath the physical in which patterns exist and from which physical conditions arise. A potentiality to a particular condition may be involved. The root cause of conditions could lie deep in some subatomic field on which the activities of the mind play an important part. Emotional effects could thus become causes. The underlying pattern of energy is obviously very complex, but it has been postulated that the whole complexity attached to the personality is contained in a very small portion of the anatomy. It may be possible by means of the instrument to discover not only what condition exists, but its cause, which may be very complex. Because the energy imbalance and not the disorder itself is being determined, for this reason the techniques of the SE-S plus are eschewed at the present time (in the U.S. at least) by the health professionals as being unorthodox.

Investigators relate that the SE-S plus obliterates space when space signifies a measure of distance. But space is not empty. It is filled with color, sound, and vibration. The SE-S plus seems to annihilate space-distance, but in reality it appears to use the life-giving potentials in space for IDF balancing.

The experimenters with the SE-S plus report it deals with effects far more fundamental than the physical since all matter is ultimately vibration. One conclusion to be reached is that well-being is the result of harmony within the complex system of resonating vibration involved in the organic structure of the body.

In the final analysis however a growing body of scientific evidence is stating that we may be composed of nothing but energy in constant transformation. It is thus easier to understand how subtle non-physical, energetic influences such as emotions and thoughts may have a direct influence on our physical functioning, just as our physical functioning may have an effect on our emotional and mental experiences. Similarly, once we understand what produces the radiant IDF emanations from our bodies, it may be clearer why these emanations should reveal something about the state of our functioning.

Researchers conclude that the chief aim of all methods directed at helping improve any condition should be directed toward the preservation, restoration and regeneration of the subtle biofield energies which may effect the electrical potential of the organism... Investigations into the nature of mind, energy and matter may prove to be one of the most profound discoveries of the 20th Century. The SE-S plus is at the forefront of a new era of technology and human consciousness. Its potential may be the potential of your own mind.

SUMMARY OF SE-5 INTRINSIC DATA FIELD ANALYZER OPERATING PRINCIPLES AND MECHANISMS

The SE-S plus INTRINSIC DATA FIELD ANALYZER is based on the premise that everything which exists emits and absorbs energy at specific vibrations. Vibrations or rates of oscillation appear to be the common denominator which describes the various states of energy from matter to thoughts. Rates of vibration can reveal what is occurring in any energy field. Vibrational energies can be measured and appear to be altered by instruments designed to neutralize abnormal or enhance normal vibrational patterns.

The SE-S plus INTRINSIC DATA FIELD ANALYZER operating mechanism can be explained in terms of known laws of physics.

1. Everything that exists is fundamentally an energy field which contains vibrational information about the contents of that field. All fields involve IDFs.

2. The interchange of matter and energy in a subtle information field can be measured in terms of wave form and amplitude.

3. The content of a wave field is based on its amplitude, wavelength and energy.

4. Every substance has a resonance which will provide increased energy proportional to its being stimulated at its resonant energy or conversely less energy if stimulated with energy opposite its resonant vibration.

The SE-S plus INTRINSIC DATA FIELD ANALYZER electronic mechanisms operate through a unique integrated circuit chip system which converts word and numerical commands into subtle informational fields. The instrument analyzes input signals from a given sample and compares them against baseline standards to determine the amplitude strength of desirable or undesirable vibrations. From this analysis an output broadcast signal is selected which may neutralize, strengthen or balance subtle energies. This process is accomplished through a series of steps:

1. Subtle radiation containing energy information from a sample is input to the translator circuit of the SE-S plus.

2. Information is entered into the computer.

3. Numerical or word commands are converted by the computer into a binary code called ASCII (standard language of computers.)

4. The ASCII code is sent to the SE-S plus translator circuits.

5. ANALYSIS: The collective information from the input sample (step 1) and the entered instructions from the computer (step 2) are then modulated at a specific amplitude wave form into one signal for analysis.

6. A resonating signal pulsed at 7.1304 Hertz is sent to a high gain amplifier designed especially to amplify IDF signals that researchers report are supportive to the overall energy field of the sample being analyzed.

7. BALANCING: The resonating signal is driven into antenna coils that output IDFs when the SE-S plus is in the balance output mode. The process is reported to employ gravitational-like energies to return the energy signal to the sample.

8. The output signal modulation appears to initiate a reduction in the difference between input and output. The modulation continues until the instrument indicates equilibrium between the actual measure and the operator's desired measure. The process is similar to that of a tuning fork or turning a thermostat to the appropriate setting.

NOTE: The SE-S plus, although containing electronic circuitry and components, does not function according to known electronic or electromagnetic mechanisms. Rather than cycles per second or Hertz resonance the SE-S plus operates with geometric resonance or pattern amplification. Information entered into the SE-S plus computer serves to tune into patterns of energy similar to morphogenic fields existing as a blueprint in the prephysical state prior to manifestation of physical phenomena.

Manufacturers of IDE instruments are not allowed to make claims. The SES plus INTRINSIC DATA FIELD ANALYZER is an experimental device to be used for research purposes only. No claims are made for the diagnosis or treatment of disease. It is the responsibility of each researcher to make their own conclusion.

CONCEPTS

IDF research, as with any discipline is based on certain tenets, principles, postulates and assumptions. Some of the more important ones are noted below and serve as a conceptual aid in conducting your research experiments.

• The law of life is motion, a rhythmic cyclic pulsation of energy which tends to preserve and restore balance and harmony. Subtle information is innate intelligence.

- All objects have natural frequencies of vibration.

- Disorders are altered functions and the natural response to strain and stress or imbalance. Altered function is nothing more than a change in vibration caused by the source of stress --whether chemical, mechanical, germ, etc. Sources of stress such as germs also have characteristic vibrations of their own.

- The application of the right energies may neutralize stressors and change altered function because all objects have the tendency to return to their original patterns if given the opportunity.

- Objects can either absorb or reflect energy vibrations according to the need.

- Changes in vibration of one part of the field can effect changes in the entire biofield as the whole and the parts are inter-related.

- As all parts of a biofield are interrelated, researchers report that it is important to: neutralize all negative or interfering energies (stressors) in the system; balance or re- establish the normal vibrations of the whole; in addition to the specific problem or imbalance.
Stressors become a problem only when the biofields natural balance is disturbed.

- The greater the harmony between the universal mind and the individual mind, the more rapidly the biofield or specific conditions can be normalized. Mind and matter are interrelated. A change in one results in a change in the other. Attitude is most important as energy follows thought. Thought is affected by the energy contained in matter. Frequency is thought in action.

- Being able to measure the presence of a particular energy rate or signal allows one to observe changes in that signal resulting from application of balancing energy, be it from allopathic, homeopathic, radionic, laying-on-of-hands or other sources of therapy.

• Researchers report being able to differentiate between signals from normal or healthy tissue and from diseased or potentially abnormal tissue. Obviously, when measuring human signals, the healthy energy rates would be present to a normal degree, while the abnormal signals would be absent or read very low.

• Where abnormal signals are present, the healthy signals are generally weak. It is reported that when abnormal signals are corrected, the healthy signals return to a normal level. Conversely, when healthy body signals return to normal levels, most abnormal signals tend to decrease.

• The imbalanced or disease-like signals appear to be reduced by application of proper balancing energy. The research charts and rate book numbers for conditions show instrument settings to signal-process the energy from the subtle bodies to provide experimental balancing energy.

• Tunings are also available for healthy signals to allow experiments to either boost or balance their amplitudes where the presence of imbalanced signals or pathogens appear to have reduced the normal readings.

• Researchers claim to be able to detect the presence of abnormal radiations in the subtle body signals using instruments, and to measure the intensity of such imbalances. The amplitudes of healthy body signals are claimed to be sensed in a similar manner.

• Where imbalanced energy is present, researchers have reported correcting such imbalance by application of the listed energy numbers for the conditions or organs and tissue involved. Analysis after such subtle body balancing has shown the correction of the energy imbalance to have taken place.

- Our intent and concentration of our attention on the research question and balancing rate is of primary consideration in IDF experiments. The SE-S plus detects and amplifies our thoughts or intent. The instrument helps, to focus, to collect and hold conscious, unconscious and super conscious energies. Because energy follows thought, as you think so shall it come to pass. We just have to be in alignment with the purpose of our efforts.

- The more knowledge we have of a particular subject matter the more clarity in our intent.

Applications - Se-5 Biofield Spectrum Analyzer

Experimental research with the SE-5 BIOFIELD SPECTRUM ANALYZER is an ongoing concern and new research applications are being developed every day by hundreds of researchers using SE-5 instrumentation.

Experimental analysis and balancing research with subtle energy instrumentation has been reportedly used to:
- Analyse the subtle energy of any objects, thoughts, emotions, relationships or environments and to send corrective signal into its Biofield.
- Measure subconscious reactions to questions.
- Identify and balance interfering emotional and mental energies.
- Detect and balance excessive and deficient subtle energies in a field.
- Test for compatibility and sensitivity to foods, products, supplements, persons and environments.
- Detect and neutralise subtle effects of pollutants, impurities and residues in foods, water garden products and household environments.
- Clear and program crystals, gems and jewellery.
- Balance energy meridians, points and auric energies.

- Locate and release energy blockages and stress factors which may lead to pain.
- Balance right and left side energy fields for efforts in super learning and performance.
- Analyse subtle energy correlation with various states and conditions of health and wellbeing.
- Analyse subtle energy field effects of various therapeutic interventions.
- Test and balance relationships, business and personal compatibilities.
- Program for self-image, self-esteem, confidence and personal growth.
- Neutralise barriers to transpersonal growth and to program affirmations and attitudes.
- Analyse and balance performance factors in achieving sports, business and personal goals.
- Locate precious metals, lost objects, artifacts, missing persons, and conduct investigations.
- Potentization, energetic duplications and replication of substances.
- Analyse potential investment opportunities, sales prospect proposals, and strategic planning.
- Troubleshooting mechanical problems and measuring quality control factors in products and schematics.

FOR EXPERIMENTAL RESEARCH PURPOSES ONLY
DESCRIPTIONS USED ARE SUBTLE ENERGY
REFERENCES AND NOT THE
ACTUAL PHYSICAL CONDITION.
(c) HUMAN SERVICES DEVELOPMENT CENTER

I was first was introduced to the SE-5 by a psychologist who used an SE-5 for her work and had great success with it and the years that have followed have been unbelievable in creating better health and harmony for me my family and my clients.

The following are some of the experiences.

1. A lady in Phoenix used to physically shake all the time when she was at home and only very little when she went out to town.

On checking the home in the whole place there were all the symptoms of an aged person who was suffering from a heart disease and extreme fear.

We balanced this energy out and everything settled down and even the owner's hyperactive cats calmed and slept more. Her shakes diminished and she was able to sleep better. On checking out with the Real Estate agent from whom she bought the old timber home, the new owner deduced the disruptive energy must have come from the long time previous owners who were very fearful and suffering from old age and heart problems.

2. A lady in Los Angeles sent me some Polaroid photos and hair samples as requested but would not divulge what was going on with her medically or energetically.

In the scan using the SE-5 it was apparent and imbalances came up many times that she had the deadly disease of AIDS and on telling her that it was in the subtle energies and may not be in the physical. This did not mean that she had AIDS or that it couldn't be cured.

She confirmed she was HIV positive and had only been given a certain time to live. Naturally she was very scared, as her boyfriend had just died of it.

As she was going back to the doctors for another test in two weeks she asked me to do what ever I could to help her. I had not had the SE-5 for very long and so said I would do my best and scanned her whole body /mind for imbalances and rebalanced them. She also purchased all the vitamins/minerals that showed up as an imbalance and took them internally and meditated daily to cut the stress levels.

At the two weeks I waited with baited breath for her to call me. She phoned and said the doctors are scratching their heads and saying they must have mis-diagnosed, as they had to give her a clean bill of health.

She was rechecked a month later and pronounced cured by the specialists. This is now many years ago and she is still healthy. Unfortunately she wanted to keep it a secret from her friends whom she felt would be upset that she could not afford to help them get well too.

3. My own motor car was developing rust and on balancing the car back to its original IDF's the rusting stopped and the car runs much better as if it was new.

4. A lady in Western Australia had an automatic car and could not get up the hill to her driveway. I took a Polaroid photo of the car and balanced it back to the original IDF's and next morning the car rushed up the hill with renewed vigour. I was astonished to say the least. Three weeks later the car was driven to the repair shop to be checked over. The mechanic came out and asked us who towed the car in and did not believe that it had been driven in until talking to his own manager who saw us drive in. Apparently the whole automatic dropped out on his floor when he undid the bolts and he showed us the mess.

5. A client in San Francisco who had many tests by many medical practitioners said she was still feeling very poorly. On scanning the subtle bodies it came up as candida which she had been tested for but had not shown up. She had the tests done again and it showed up and was treated accordingly.

6. Client in Indiana sent me a hair sample and I phoned her two hours later to say that it looked as though she had the subtle energies of cancer showing up and that she was bleeding internally. She agreed and said she was trying to get into hospital to have this operated on to stop the bleeding but there was a large waiting list. She asked me to try and stop the bleeding in the appropriate area and this was done successfully within two hours. She did have the operation at a later time but as she put it she could have bled to death waiting for the operation.

7. As babies cannot tell us what the problem is to scan the subtle energies and to see what could be wrong is very rewarding! An infection in the middle ear that was missed was important.

8. I have been able to pick what area has compatible energies for me to look for a home or apartment to live in. You can find out on a map what cross streets to have a closer look at.

9. A little girl close to me one morning kept falling down and was in obvious pain and the mother called me to observe and to ask me should she take her to the hospital.

Immediately after it was seen the distress she was in it was arranged for her to go to the hospital and it was going to take some time for the blood tests to come back.

A scan covers the full body and an hour to two hours of time. I stated in the energies it looked like rheumatic fever and started balancing her on the mothers consent. The tests came back very similarly with Guillian Barre' syndrome as the cause which are both similar diseases and the only main difference being according to my books, one originally from England and one from France and both had very similar symptoms energetically.

The mother was told her daughter could be in hospital many months and she was home in under a week.

10. At a haunted house we took photographs both front and back of the house and a couple of photos where the ghostly appearances occurred. We were able to trace down accurately the lady in question who had died there, her date of birth, the age she died etc. and sent her to be with her loved ones in the light. The apparitions stopped from that day and the house energies according to the owners became much more settled.

11. Many sports people who are taking vitamin/minerals have been scanned to see what their bodies can absorb and what vitamins/ minerals are missing and in what order and time the substances can be assimilated.

12. Affirmations are accurately designed to fit in with your energy grids for maximum benefit.

13. Business checks by owners as to whom are the persons who need to be watched more closely when pilfering is going on.

There are many incredible stories like this and too many too narrate here, as it would take too many pages to give credence to it. I am still totally blown away with the miracles I have seen and done with this

SE-5. I am convinced that the SE-5 is only limited by the operator and his imagination / ability / solving skills.

An SE-5 can be ordered from Living from Vision PO Box 1530 Stanwood WA 98292 or Ph 1-800-758-7836 and tell Don Paris who is a excellent operator and trainer of the SE-5. You can read all about the SE-5 in his book Regaining Wholeness through the Subtle Dimensions on his website. www.healingconnection.com.au or www.se-5.com for more information.

STRESS /TENSION

Stress and tension are considered to be the most major contributing factor in at least 75 per cent of all illness and in 11 of 12 main causes of death in the world today!
We need a certain amount of stress to challenge us, motivate us, keep us healthy, and carry us to peak of fitness and performance. And yet one degree beyond the healthy amount we begin to slide into being unhealthy.

We experience stress and tension in many ways:
Stress induced headaches
Stress induced backaches
Stress induced muscle aches
Stress induced joint pain
Stress induced skin rashes
Stress induced sleep disturbance
Stress induced stomach aches
Stress induced depression
Stress induced sexual function
The human senses are on duty 24 hours of the day scanning inside us and outside of us for signs of stress. When something out of the ordinary happens these senses or subconscious mind alert the brain in lightning fast speed so we can get out of danger if there is some. The brain alerts the glands which in turn releases chemicals into the blood stream like adrenalins and cortisol and all systems are placed on full alert and instantly prepared for action even beyond in some circumstances what we think we are capable of. The heart begins to pound, blood pressure increases, breathing quickens, digestion

slows or stops, perspiration begins to cool the body and there is an increase of oxygenated blood to the muscles and brain.

As sophisticated as our system is, it cannot distinguish between real or imagined or excitement or joy so you could have the same reaction when you see a shark in the water swimming close to you as when you are standing at the altar waiting to say your marriage vows. Were you stressed with your knees knocking then?

Some of the major points of **Stress Management and Avoiding Burnout** according to Major Phillip Dalton of Academy of Health Sciences in Fort Sam Houston Texas are.

Stress and Tension of Change
Beginning, leaving a job, moving into or out of a home, relationship, experiencing gain or loss.

Stress and Tension of Chemical
Chemicals that cause harm to your body like caffeine, sugar, salt, diet pills, sleeping pills, and other legal-illegal chemicals. Chemicals in the environment, pesticides, exhaust fumes, paint fumes, tobacco smoke, etc.

Stress and Tension of Commuting
The factors of driving to and from work safely. In a hurry, have a time frame to destination, kids in the car, what the weather is like, argument with someone close to you.

Stress and Tension of Decision
Confronted with an important decision and not enough information or time to give it careful consideration. Some decisions do not have right or wrong answers no matter what you decide. Usually the first answer in your mind will be the right one.

Stress and Tension of Disease
Experiencing long or short-term acute or chronic illness always takes a lot of energy to cope or recover from. As stress weakens the immune system sometimes the energy required to combat disease is not available and causes more stress.

Stress and Tension of Emotion
Fears and anxieties and worry never solved any problem. Complaining is contagious and takes a tremendous amount of energy both to speak it and also to listen to it.

Stress and Tension of Environment
Response to noise, light, temperature and extremes are factors that rob us of energy.
Stress and Tension of Family
Experienced in the constant challenge of keeping relationships balanced and flowing.
Stress and Tension of Social
Attempt to balance your own needs with those of family and others.
Stress and Tension of Work
Demands placed on you at work are the number one predictor of how long you are expected to live in this country.

Choices / power points in managing stress
1.Nutrition is important. Educate yourself about food beyond whether it tastes good or not. Chew slowly and masticate the food properly before swallowing. No TV eating and no arguing and complaining, while eating breathe between each mouthful.
2.Rest is important for replenishment of energy and provides time to heal. Too much rest can be just as bad for you as not enough rest. When experiencing certain types of fatigue, change in activity is clearly superior to sleep.
3.Body maintenance (physical exercise) is imperative to stimulate metabolism, tone muscles, oxygenate the system, strengthen and tone muscles, assist digestion and peristalsis and improve the immune and lymphatic system.
4.Balance in giving is important, as life is a system of balances. A fulltime caretaker who only gives to others all the time is in a situation of imbalance and will eventually give too much out or crash out.
5.Only do for others that they cannot do for themselves as if they can do it and you do it for them it will only make them weaker and they won't have any pride in themselves. Remember to teach them to fish and they can feed themselves and not need to rely on anyone.
6.Don't say yes when your gut says no!
7.Keep a diary and write things down as it has been proven that one is more organised and three times likely to succeed.
8.Get off automatic pilot and think about your choices before decision making.

A smile is all it takes

It is most important for all people to realise that in this world that if one is less fortunate than I **there but for the grace of God go I** so judgement is not an option. A smile never costs anything and some of the greatest healings today are affected by a smile.

I used to walk every day down to get the paper and every day an old man used to walk past me, bent over as though the whole world was on his shoulders. Every morning I would say good morning and keep moving until about two months later he stopped me and said, "What's good about it?" I stated it was a beautiful day and it was good to be alive and walked on. He said "Poppycock!" as I walked away.

The next day after my greeting he asked me to stay and talk for a while so we sat down on a street seat and he was full of complaints about his family and his grandchildren who were making so much noise he felt he was being driven to distraction. After a while of listening to all this painful heartfelt verbiage I asked him what he was like as a child and was he just as vibrant and loud as his grandchildren? He answered that he had given his parents a really hard time and when he mentioned that I stated it looked like those grandchildren were just like a chip of the old block, meaning him, so I guessed he was reaping what he sowed for his parents. He naturally had not thought about it that way, but over the next few months he became more and more close to his grandchildren.

It came to a time I had to leave and go on my yearly healing trips overseas and I told him one morning I was leaving. He was obviously very distressed, that I asked him to do me a favor and do as I had done for him and keep smiling at people who looked like life was getting them down and talk, to help lighten their load, to which he promised.

I had great joy in driving past six months later to see the same old man seated on the park bench talking to another man rather animatedly enjoying the day.

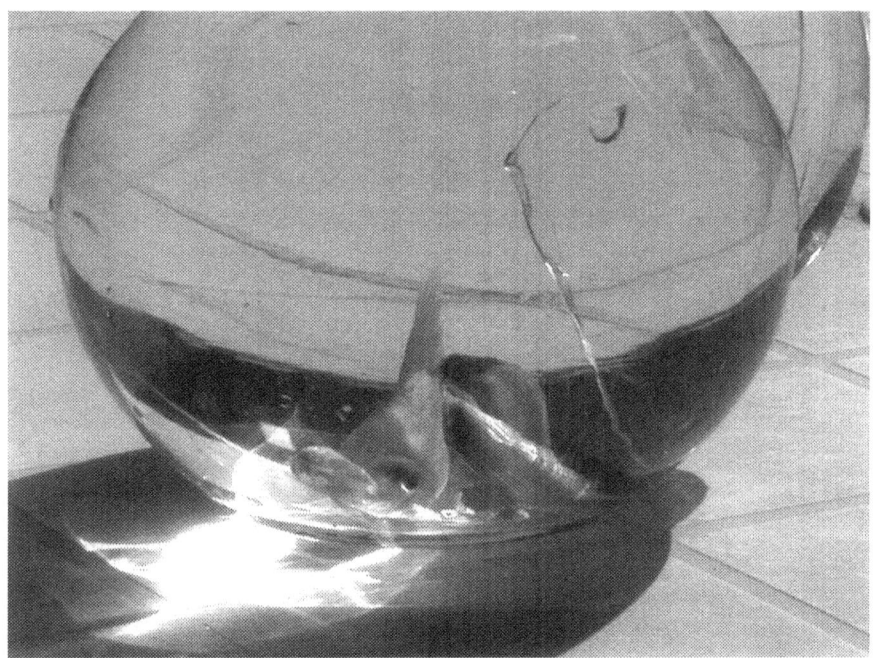

1.Goldies world is cracked but he too has an etheric friend

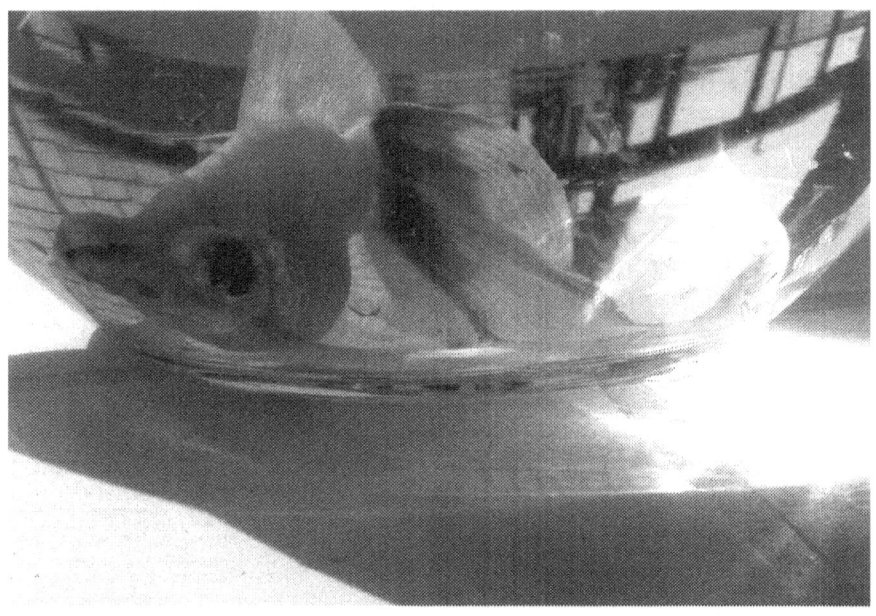

2.Boy am I stuffed! It's a jungle out there!

This little fish was black once and once when I was really unhappy I stated to those who were listening that I was really angry and believed they were not listening to or helping me with my projects. I stated that the way things were going I had as much chance of being realised as this little black fish turning gold. It started turning gold within two weeks and in a month it was as it looks now. Oops! Be careful what you say.

Talking to your subconscious and inner creative mind for answers follows.

INNER-CREATIVE MIND, (Positive)
SUBCONCIOUS MIND, (Disruptive Programming)

TALKING OR GETTING ANSWERS FROM YOUR INNER CREATIVE MIND.

It is usually best to get a friend or a Hypnotherapist to take you through for the first time. It is suggested if you have not done any self healing work on yourself in seminars before that you get a professional therapist to help you with this until you become proficient. When you practice and get good at this method you can get answers to things like, is this food good for me? or is this person telling the truth? and similar.

1. Establish yourself in a quiet safe place, making yourself comfortable preferably sitting up so you do not fall asleep and by uncrossing your arms and legs so you will not cramp or get pins and needles from lack of circulation. When you feel sure that you won't be disturbed physically and mentally, breathe deeply and slowly while projecting your mind into your heartspace usually located in your chest area in the aproximate area of your heart or heart energy center.

2. Ask to talk to your subconcious or inner-creative mind. They are different aspects of the mind but are one and the same and it is like talking to a part of yourself! When addressing your inner-creative mind, in this case a positive part of the no restriction simple part in your mind that only knows black or white (no grey areas) and is programmed by feelings, emotions, environment, conditioning,

racial and family DNA even automatic patterns before birth. It takes patterns from your mother and father like blood temperature, breathing, skin color, heartbeat, eye focusing etc. It does not know what is right or wrong, just what is.

3.Establish in your mind a friendship - love bond and talk to your mind as a true and trusted friend telling it you are needing answers by saying, "I am now an adult and I wish to take more responsibility. I wish to make changes to my life and make things easier for my conscious and inner-creative mind, so less energy is spent physically or mentally in my life to gain happy, harmonious positive results. Many decisions were made when I was younger to automatically protect me when I did not understand. I now wish to re-look at some of those decisions as I am now an adult and look at things differently. Do you understand? Are you willing to help me release my old fears and seed memories?" Try to get a feeling.
Usually a warm feeling indicates a positive answer and a cold or yucky feeling may be a no.
Everyone is different as I have even had a child say she saw beautiful butterflies for a yes answer and cold waterfalls for a no answer.

4.Establish a yes/no answer response with your forefinger responding on either hand. It depends on your preferance as to whether you are left handed or right.

After laying your hand on your stomach so you can see your fingers on either hand move ask.
a:" Inner-creative mind please answer me with a lifting of my finger strongly, preferably my forefinger on right hand, when you wish to answer me with a yes answer." Repeat this at least three times as communication must be clear and if the response from the finger is not strong enough ask for it to be stronger and intensify the lifting of the finger until you are satisfied with the communication.

b:"Inner-creative mind if you wish to communicate a no answer keep my hands and fingers still." As before at least three times for clarity. "Do you understand?" Wait for the answer with the lifting of your finger. When it lifts say "thank you for talking to me," and go ahead with the next stage. If no response at all, sometimes a response can be obtained by merely asking for a yes response.

5."I now want to work on the project of _____" and imagine, visualise, sense, and know, of a big picture or video screen in front of you in this space in your chest called your heart room or heart space. Have your screen in front at about 22 degrees above the floor, about seven normal steps up, of where you are standing in the middle of the room. Split the screen into two picture screens although joined together. The left screen is the present / past screen and used for portraying you like an actor on the screen sensing /seeing / feeling negative / disruptive energies you don't /didn't like or didn't want to have happen in your life. The right screen is for a positive present or how and what you want need in your life to be happy now and in the future.

Working with your inner-creative mind.

6.Relax into it with if it works it works attitude and do not try to force anything.
Visualize with as much emotion as possible on the present / past left screen what is happening in your life now or lately with what you haven't liked. When you really feel the negative emotions / memories, visualize this project clearly with all the negative / disruptive emotion attached to it and when you feel you are satisfied there is no more to sense, then draw a black cross diagonally across the screen with force as though you are stamping a stamp on paper or closing the lid on a trash can of rubbish. Set a violet fire at the bottom and round the sides of the picture ready to contain and burn all the negative emotions and feelings away.

7.Now visualize on the right screen with as much emotion as possible how you want your life to be in the future with this project. Visualize sense with **emotion!** You as an actor are changing and decreeing that you are going to have a peaceful harmonious life in the future. If you are having trouble bringing up positive emotion then think back to a time when you may have experienced happiness previously in your life concerning this project even if it was only for five minutes similar to a birthday, Christmas being given a gift, a time singing, a wonderful childhood friend. If you having trouble remembering anything positive no matter how small, imagine what it would be like to be successful in this project, see / sense, imagine, pretend yourself being happy, content, prosperous, healthy, harmonious, enjoying your success. Remember it takes more energy to frown than to smile and if the subconscious mind does not know the difference between real or imagined then you are your own jet pilot in this exercise.

8.When the feeling of success is there in the right screen, concentrate on the left screen and burn and transform all your negative pictures, feelings, emotions away with the violet flame saying "This is the old me, not the new me!"

With your left screen now vacant leave it with your hand written flowing golden letters glowing brightly like neon lights with the words of peace, love, joy and harmony. Let these words fade into the screen.

9.Ask your inner-creative mind now if it understands, "Do you understand that the picture on the left screen which has now been transformed or burnt away was not what I have wanted in my life?" Get a yes / no answer. Be specific and uncomplicated with your talking to the inner creative mind as though you are talking to a slow thinking child and or a double personality of yourself that is unsure and not feeling safe.

Remember the picture that remains on the right screen is the future and always is what you want in your life, so you ask your mind to help, "Will you help me to attain positive results to this project as quickly as possible without any ill effects to me. Thankyou," if appropriate answer.

10.Then ask "Do you understand?" and get a yes / no response. If no, repeat with more detail. Get if possible a yes-answer.

11.Next: Assure your subconcious mind, "I do not wish to take away any of your power. I just wish to redirect the energies to have less tension, be able to relax more and do more with less energy expended so we are both happy and creative."

12. Ask,"Inner-creative mind, will my conscious mind be able to understand the pictures to make change?" Yes / no and if no, "Do you want to talk to me?" yes / no. Get the yes / no flow going, it's like a rusty tap, it's sometimes a little hard to turn on. If still no, ask "Will you please release away all disruptive energy on all levels over the next few weeks in dream therapy so we may attain our goal which is on the right screen?" Yes / no answer. If no ask more questions and quietly cajole to get yes answer if possible.

If yes answer, then be prepared to become the actor /actress in your own life on the screen.
Say "Inner creative mind, please show me clearly and concisely in picture / feeling form on the left screen at the front, what has happened in this lifetime that was so devastating, so hurtful, so disappointing, that you changed the energy, protected me from having similar experiences again, so I wouldn't be emotionally hurt again. I thank you for protecting me but now I am an adult, I can understand more, and wish now to judge for myself. Please show me the pictures clearly with intensity in the order I am able to handle emotionally," and watch/sense on the screen as forgotten parts of your prior life unfolds.

Note:Be patient and let your mind drop through the fear and into the blackness if you can as you have done it all before so there is nothing in your life you have not experienced before, some emotion can come up as an old emotional hurts come up, **so be prepared! Keep some tissues handy**. You may generally see yourself much younger than you are now. If the picture is not clear ask to see more clearly, and you can always ask for the inner-creative mind to **intensify the picture** so you can recognise why your subconscious in its wisdom has taken action in wanting to protect you from going though the trauma again, stopped this emotional energy from coming into your life, this reward or whatever. Some correlation will be between this old picture of your life and the new positive picture you want in your life. When you have the whole scene clearly say "Inner-Creative Mind," and explain simply to your mind why this happened and as now you are an adult you no longer need protection from this as you now understand. Expain to your mind using A.B.C. as follows:

Using this technique I was able to see why money /prosperity never came into my life prior to this exercise as I was shown pictures which I had forgotten. Every time I was given something of value there was always a very emotional time as most of the things I loved when I was young were shortly after taken away, sold or broken. To protect me from all this sorrow my subconcious mind virtually stopped the energy of people giving me things to stop me being emotionally hurt. After doing this cycle I bought a lotto ticket and won $25 and actually picked up money dropped on the ground which I had never done before. This was a big imbalance which has now been resolved, thank God.

A.Tell your mind why that can't or shouldn't happen again.You are bigger, stronger, an adult now, etc. Remember that to re-experience a childhood problem is like facing up to a 60 foot angry giant in your adult life. Remember you were looking at kneecaps when tiny so have patience with yourself as what you are trying to look at was an emotive time. Answers can be slow in coming and one time I did not appear to be getting anywhere and then the next two nights I had dreams about it all. If at all unsure seek professional help.

B. Explain how you would rather experience life than be cut off from experiencing life.

C. You are older now and can accept the challenge of living in the now. Find something about any negative picture you are able to laugh about and you will find it changes the energy quicker.

13.Put a black cross diagonally across the screen of your own left screen memory and burn / transmute all emotion away with a violet flame. Any disruptive picture on the left side which was your negative memories shown to you by your subconcious mind must be cleared. Thank your mind when this is done and then write in a flowing handwriting with your own hand, peace, love, joy, harmony across the screen in large glowing golden letters and let it fade into your mind back to a blank screen.

ALWAYS USE POSITIVE REINFORCEMENT

14. For positive reinforcement on the left screen concentrate on a time about the same time, same age as the negative picture just shown to you, maybe a few days before or after the nasties happened.

A time of happiness, fulfillment, joy, harmony even if it was for five minutes, a birthday or Christmas feeling the feelings before or after disaster struck. Bring them into your body. Imagine how you would have liked the outcome to have been if you are not able to get any positive feelings as though you are able to direct your own picture for life. Then going to the right-hand screen and putting those feelings into the picture you want in the future, let the left picture fade.

Many people remember a toy, pet or favorite thing during this time that they have long since forgotten.

15. Ask Inner-Creative Mind or subconcious mind whatever you prefer it to be called, - "Are there any more pictures for me to look at now?" Yes / no response. Continue to see all the pictures one by one but don't judge yourself! You have served time to beat yourself up! Don't do it anymore! If you are a spark of God having the human experience then every time you criticize yourself you criticize God. You can ask to see the seed picture as to when all your fears really started and all subsequent fears attached to it.

When the seed emotion is released all the other emotions / pictures will usually fall over like a pack of dominoes.

16. When all pictures have been released and transmuted into light give thanks to your Inner-creative mind, ask it, "Please now let go of any disruptive energy which could stop me from obtaining the goals that I am looking towards attaining during the following weeks in dream therapy. This releasement in a manner that my concious mind and body can handle in good health." Get a yes answer that your mind will do this if possible.

17.Relive the picture of yourself now filled with loving emotion in your living painting completed to this stage of progress for you to experience or relive when you get up every morning or go to bed. Create how you would love to experience your day from morning till nighttime for the next 14 days at least allowing nothing but perfect result.

Daily Programming /Reaffirming what you want in life.
18.If any disruptive happenings still happen in following days, remember how and what you have programmed your inner-creative mind. Put all negatives /disruptive energies experienced in your life on the left screen every nightime before you go to sleep. For example, reliving the negative things that have happened during the day and feeling the negative emotions.

Then when the feelings are at their peak of intensity black cross them diagonally - and say to yourself: "Inner-Creative Mind, this is the old me, this is not the new me! I did not like nor want that to happen and will now not accept this back into my life in any form of reality."

Burn /Transmute negative disruptive energies away using the violet flame and then writing in a flowing hand in gold lettering glowing like a neon sign, peace, love, joy, and harmony on the screen and start to relive your living painting on the right screen in the next step.

For the next step it is always a great idea to think of all of the wonderful things that happened in the current day, no matter how small. Feel the state of grace the happiness and positive emotions you felt during the current day on your left screen and then infuse them into your right screen in the future. Sensing you acting out how you want to be with full feeling and emotion and then say, "This is the real me and how I want to be. " Then take the enthusiastic fantastic positive feelings /emotions over to your right future screen and ground this in. This will instruct your subconscious mind in what you get excited about and are looking forward to out of your life and will bring the 60 billion brain cells to focus on what you do want. When you feel you are finished for the session /day bring both screens together as the left screen should have faded by now. You may then take the painting for your present and future life off the screen and hang it on the wall of your heart room, preferably to the right of your screen of mind, for you to add to at a later date.

19.To do other projects in following days simply lift your living painting off and hang it on a conspicuous place on a wall at the front of your heartroom or space, cleanse the screen split into two screens and start your next project as before.
It is not a good idea to do any more than five major issues a week.

Remember if you are not sure, have not done any emotional work on yourself before in workshops, excessive emotion like fear comes up, if you are not getting anything at all, realise there could be something in your subconscious that you would not be able to understand or handle without professional help.
Don't be a martyr as this way may not be the path for you. Get a professional therapist to help you get through your blocks and barriers to a fulfilled life.

Spiritual Photos

For those of you who feel you on your own and still are not convinced that there are Masters and Angels present in our daily life, I really feel you are missing out on a beautiful mystique part in life. Therefore I am adding a small collection of photos that were given to me to share and give inspiration to those who were sick and dying. Enjoy! Let them have their own message for you.

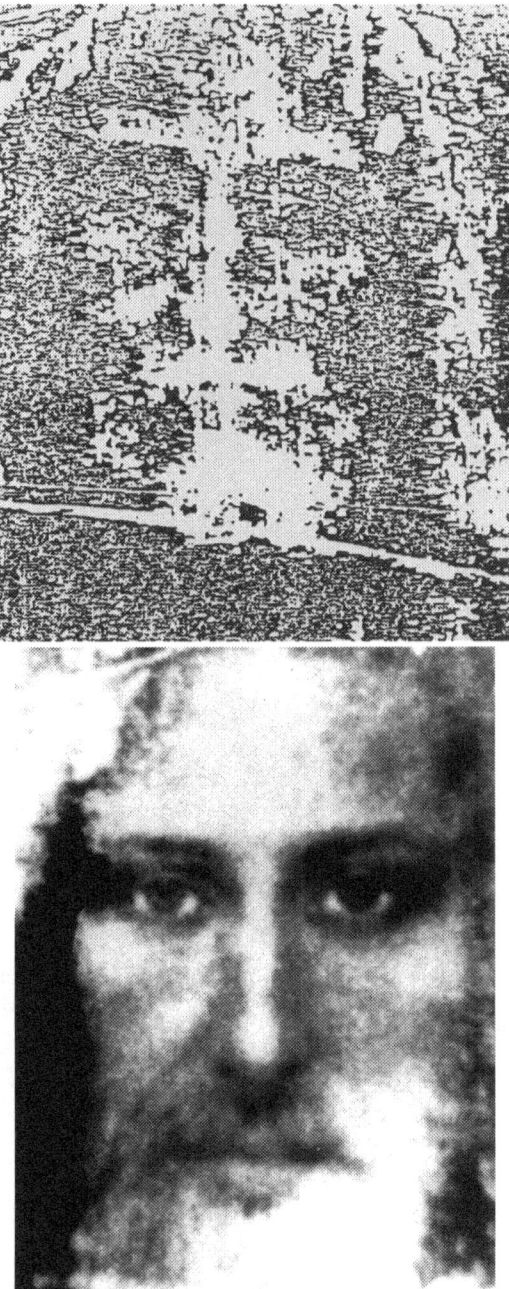

The shroud of Turin and the photo that Sathya Sai Baba blessed
and turned into color for all to see what Jesus looked like.

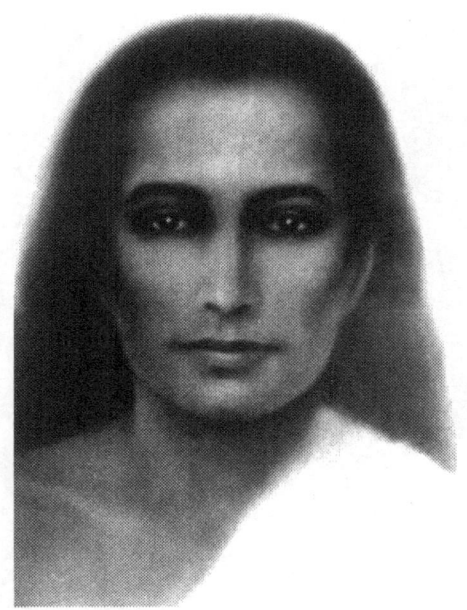

Master Barbaji (balanced man face) who is thousands of years old.

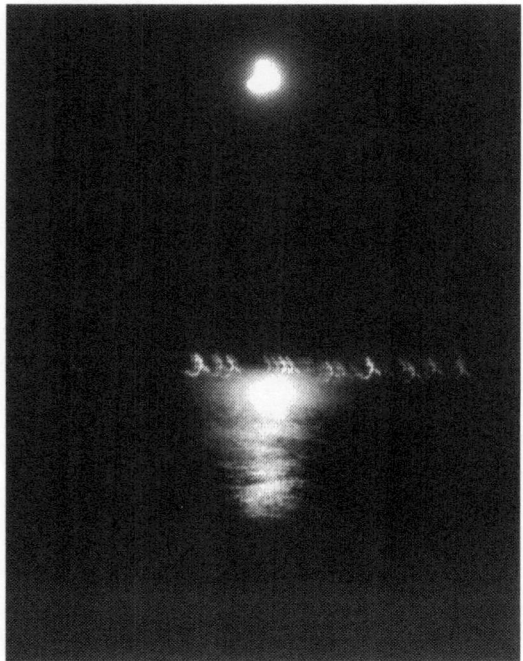

Photo of the moon while thinking of my mother who had just died
a short time before.

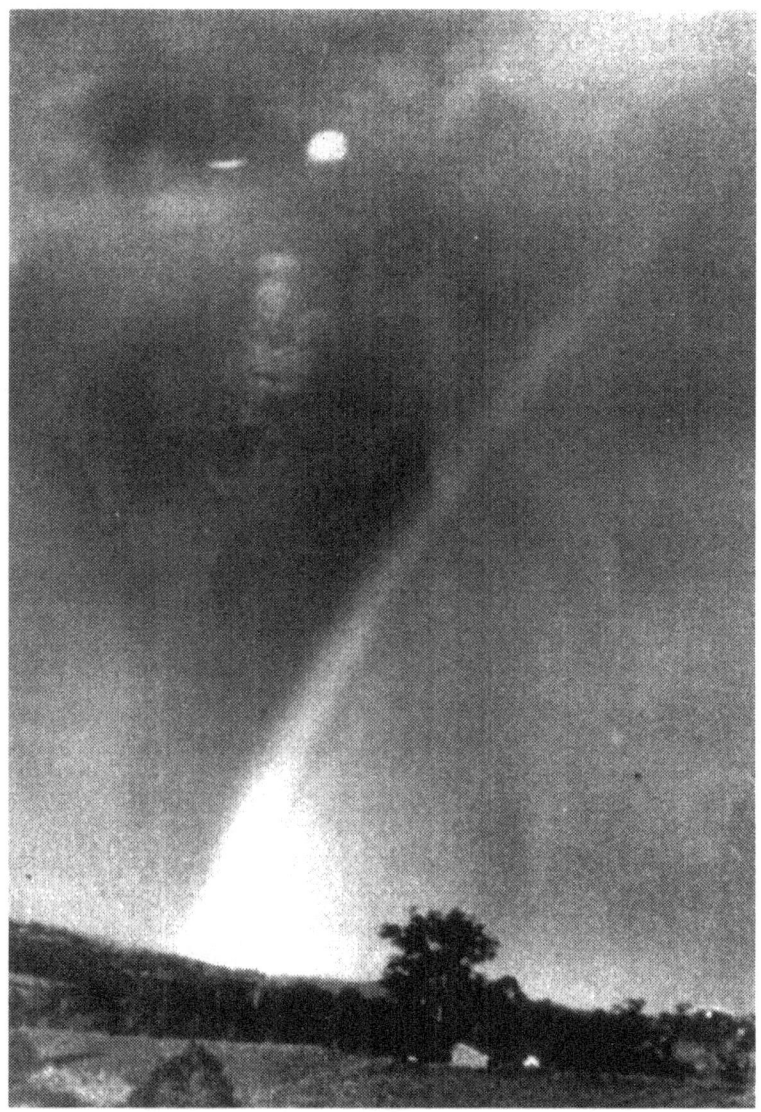

Photo of a rainbow at Yandina in Queensland Australia
Mother Mary and child to left of rainbow

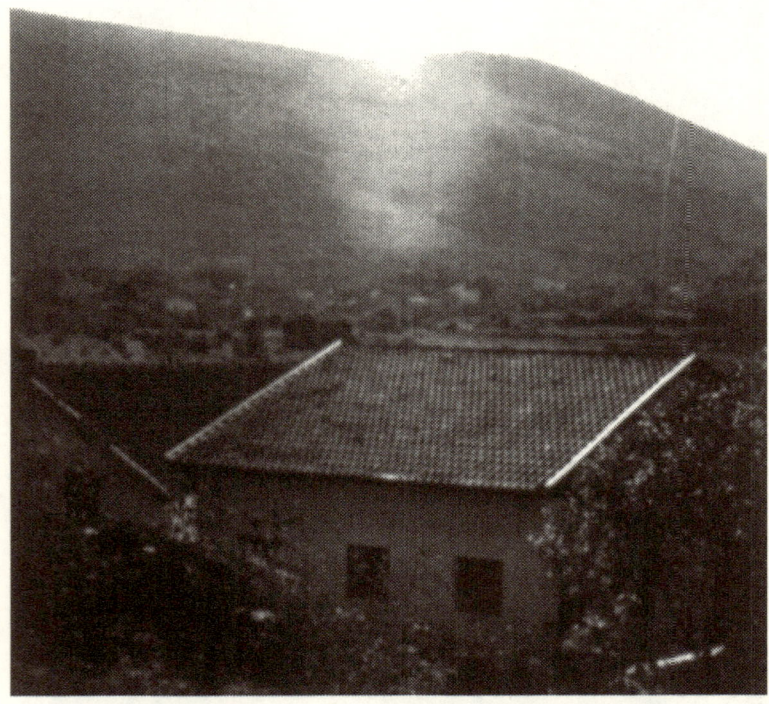

Mother Mary's appearance at Medjugorji
Apparition of Mary when she appeared to six Croatian village girls

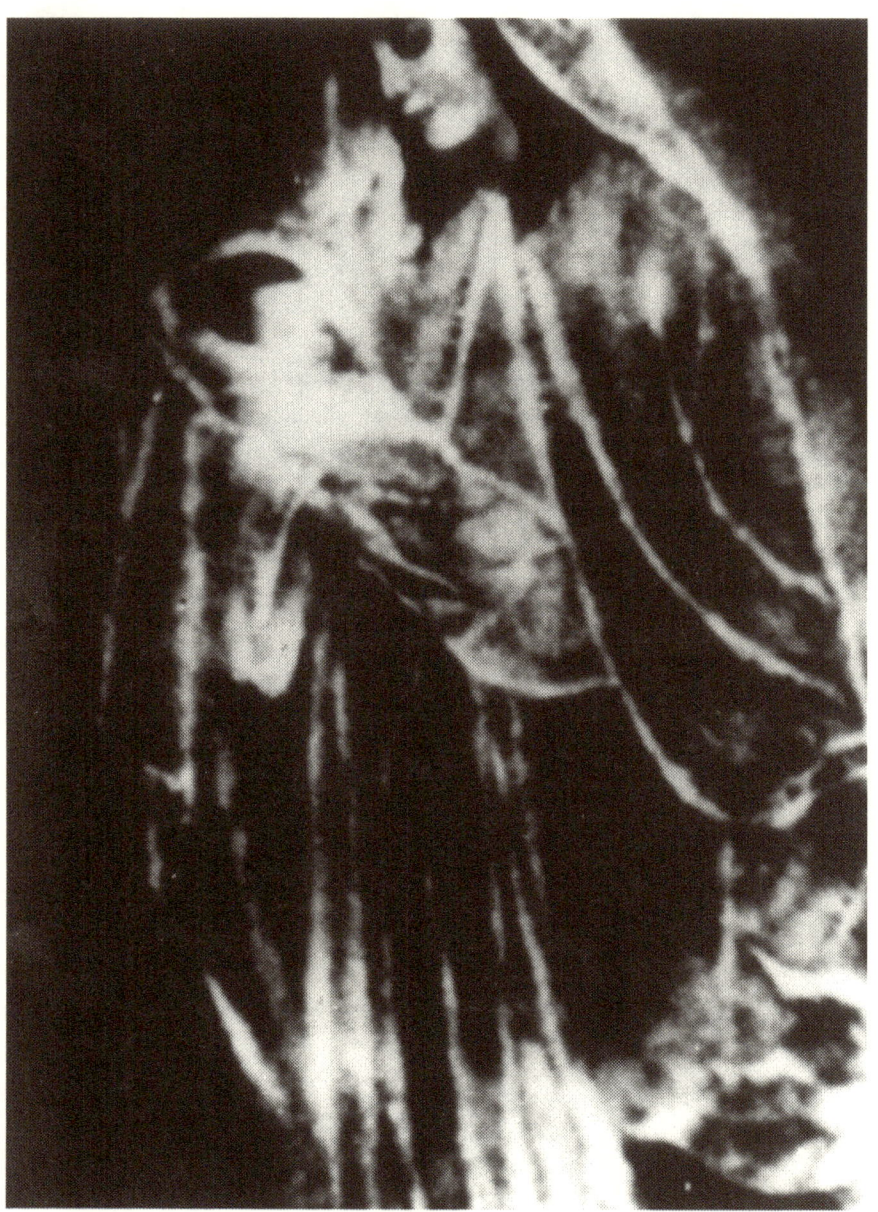

Mother and child photo in a church.

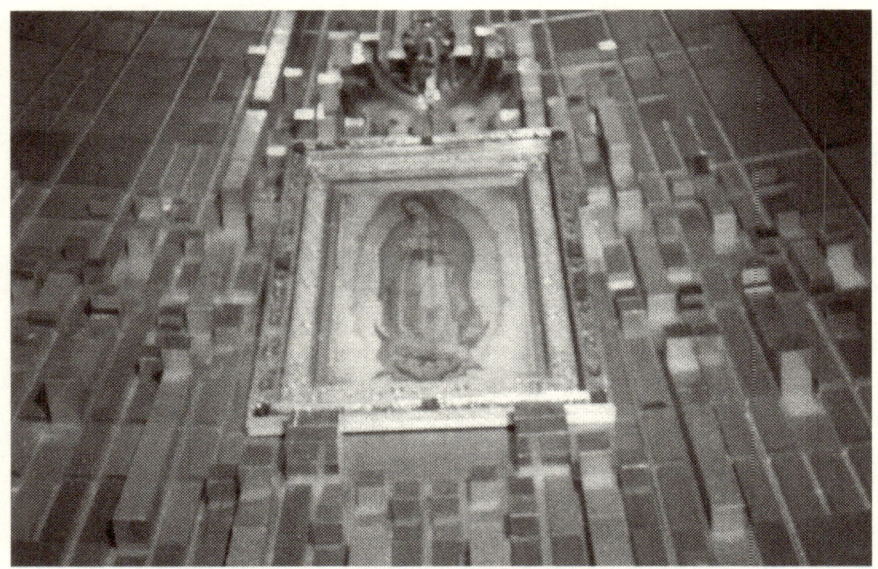

Apparition framed of The Lady of Guidalupe.
From the back of a devoted old man's poncho
For priests to take notice to build a church in Mexico City

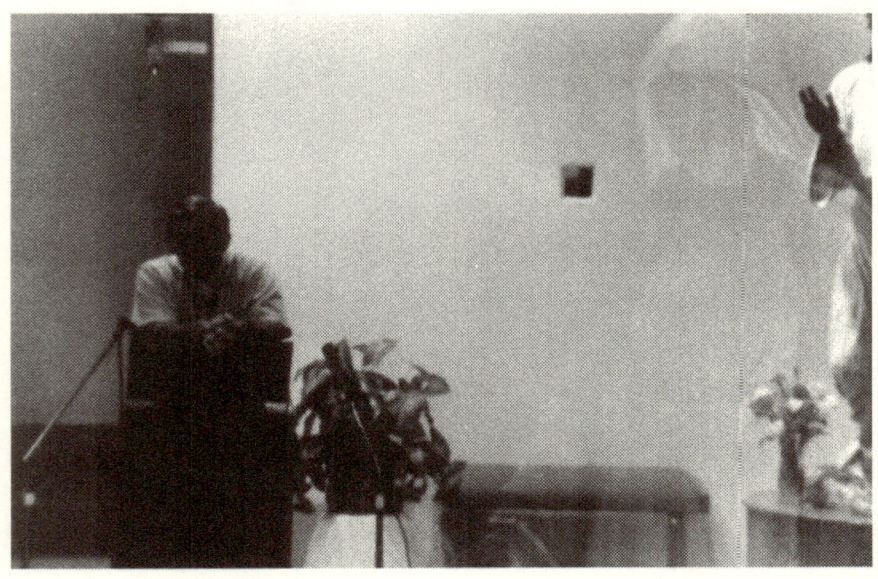

Photo taken at a Scottsdale church of Mary's Statue on right,
apparition on left of statue.

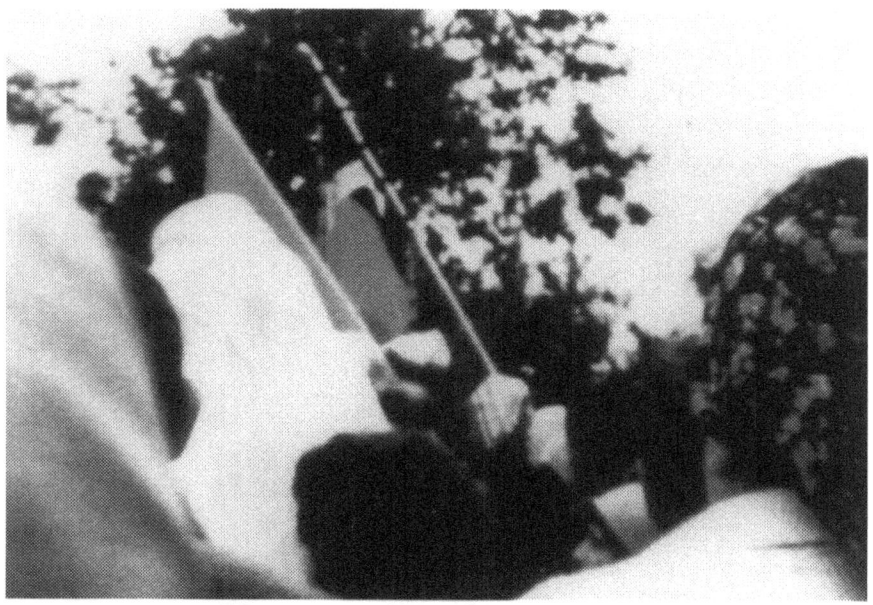

Parade in Philippines in memory of the Ghost of Mother Mary.

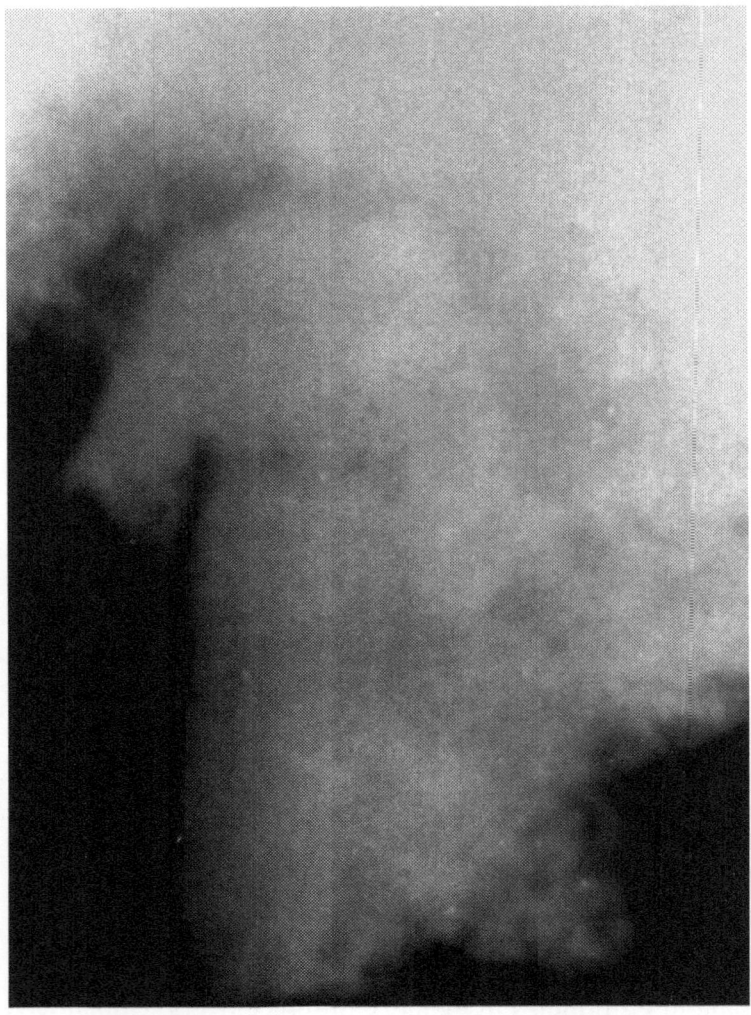

This photo was taken from a window of a plane flying between Australia and New Zealand by a religious lady who was praying for her and the others in the plane as the pilot had stated there was not much hope after the plane hit a thunderstorm. All of a sudden the storm calmed and the plane completed the trip successfully. When her film came back this was the surprise. Was a Master present to calm the tempest and answer the prayers of those on board?
We are not alone!

Epilogue

So it's now all up to you.

I would like to share with you a part of a letter written to me May 26, 1986 by none other than the courageous Shirley Mac Laine which even today is inspirational in my life.

Shirley Mac Laine

May 1986

Dear John,

These are such exciting times we live in, particularly if our points of view resonate to the light and love of God above and the light and love of the God within.

Every seemingly tragic event that occurs in our lives occurs for a reason. The reason is for the purposeful good of our own growth. If we can constantly remember that we chose to experience what we are living in our lives in order to realize the God within us, life will become glorious and the way we relate to **tragedy** alters.

My most important lesson has been to understand that there is really no such thing as reality. It is all a question of **perception**. The way we **perceive** life is everything. In other words, we are not the victims of the world we see, we are the victims of the way we **see** the world.

Therefore a positive and productive life is up to each one of us individually. **We** are our own realizers. We are our own teachers. Please understand that **you** are a God. You are love. You are light. And our free will is the path of understanding, the total realization of the God within us.

Keep your knowingness of the God within intact.

Trust yourself and trust your inherent love and light will manifest in the same way.

The kingdom of Heaven is within **you**. Make no one your master. Make no one else your idol. Make yourself all there is, and your life will become complete. You and God are one.

Much love and light from me and thank you again.

Shirley

Thank you for using your energy to purchase this book as a percentage of the proceeds will go to helping people who are less fortunate than us to get operations and healings. I really hope that you have found some information in this book that you have been able to use for the betterment of your life and I wish you all the love, success and joyful health that the Universe can offer you. The idea for this book to be written was instigated when I observed that many people ran from doctor to therapist to courses that promised the world. Most times they forgot to take back their own power, look for their own answers within and to discern the answers that lay in their everyday life. Everything in this book has been used successfully at one time or another and worked well to varying degrees.

As I do not know all your personal facts it would be impertinent for me to say these tried and trusted therapies will work for everyone. If you have any doubts no matter how slight with what I have suggested in this book as to what could or would work for you, please check with your trusted professional doctor or naturopath.

Love, Light, Joy and Laughter
John Chamberlin
The Healing Connection www.healingconnection.com.au

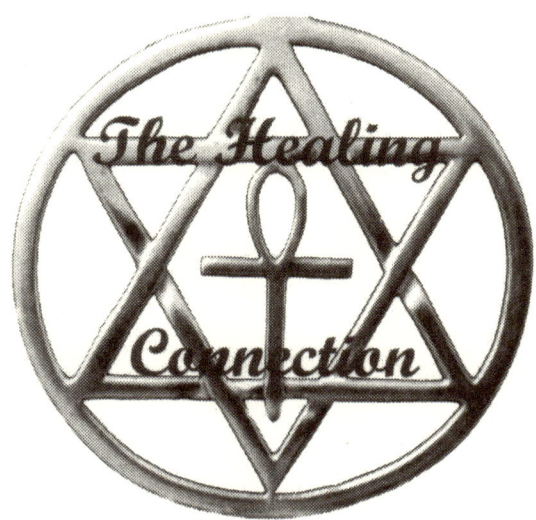

The Healing Connection Pentacle

The Pentacle symbol was shown to me in a deep meditation/prayer during a healing and manifested into the physical for me to wear.

I was informed it is representative of all known races, creeds and religions in our Universe, no soul more or less than any other is, all from the same source originally and going back to the same source eventually. All striving to attain mastership, be fully realised and complete the missions we have come in to complete, to put aside greed, graft, corruption, unbalanced health and ultimately co-exist peacefully in health, wealth, harmony and joy.

It has to start somewhere so this mission I took up not only to help my own health and that of my family but also to make a difference on the planet no matter how small. Having worked around the world many others have joined in this quest of making a positive change.

The outer circle symbolically represents the Universe and the outer bodies and five points of man, The two triangles slightly off center mean as above so below, bringing the knowledge down and ground it on this planet. It is also representative of the Jewish Star of David, the Cross, the Egyptian Ankh, Ancient Wisdom, Ancient Mysteries, the Sword of Truth, the Eternal Flame, the Eternal Spirit, and the eye of God.

Being such a small piece it is not possible to put all symbols in but they are represented in spirit.

About the Author

Clairvoyant-Medium and Spiritual Healer/Advanced Hypnotherapist/Advanced Massage-Bodywork Therapist/Reiki Master /Group Seminar Motivator Meditation Leader.

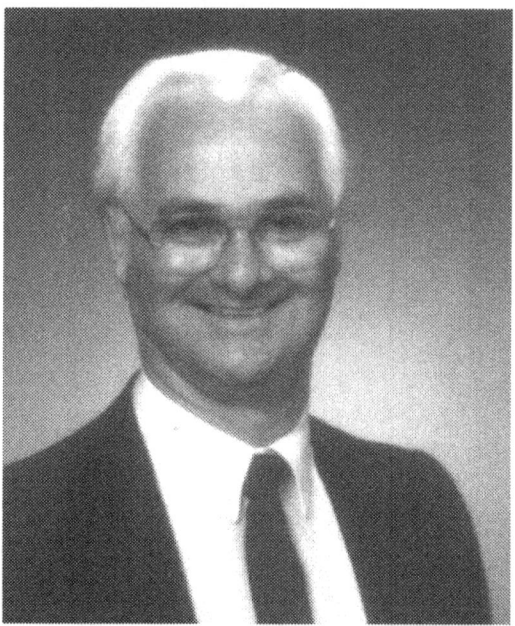

John Chamberlin has been in the field of health and healing for most of his life, in particular, full time for the last 20 years. He is known throughout the world as a leading edge motivator to encourage people to be responsible for their own bodies, to take control of their own dis-ease, destiny and dysfunction within their own conscious/ subconscious and bodily functions causing the current energy blocks to change to good health and joy.

He has been invited to speak and work in:
Australia where he operated The Tree of Life Healing Center and now for The Healing Connection in Southport, Queensland,
Second International Health /Healing Conference in Brisbane with renown Psychic Surgeons
Health and Harmony Expo in Perth in 1994,

New Zealand at the 2 nd International Healers for Peace Conference in 1990,
The Philippines, working in a missionary type of healing work with the people,
Mexico as a Spiritual Releasement Therapist,
Stockholm Sweden, at Pan Center for Health,
Copenhagen Denmark, Physiotherapy College

And has had speaking working engagements in Health and Healing for the World Renown Whole Life Expo in Los Angeles, New York, Bedford Texas, Phoenix, Tucson, Denver Colorado, etc in The United States of America,

He has been interviewed in America on:
Colorado Cable TV
Mile High TV
Manhattan Cable TV CH D-17
Paragon Cable TV CH C-16
UA Columbia TV.CH-8
Cablevision TV CV 27
Queens Pay TV CH 56
Continental TV CH 26

He is a member of:
Australian Traditional Medicine Society #0878
American National Guild of Hypnosis #G413785203
American Associated Bodywork and Massage Professionals (International Certification #101243)
Certified in Swedish Massage
Advanced Swedish Massage and Bodywork
Reiki 1, 2, 3, and Mastership
Spiritual Healing
Reflexology
Kinesiology
Advanced and Alchemy Hypnosis
Instructor Train the Trainer Basic Hypnotherapy for the National Guild of Hypnotists
Instructor in Physio Body Movement Therapies
Reverend and Healing Priest

John Chamberlin is an Australian citizen born and raised in a New Zealand farming community in a dysfunctional family. His first recollection of healing ability was when as small child a bird flew into a closed window of the house, fell lifeless to the ground and was pronounced dead by John's mother and sister. After the others had left, seeing the beauty of this little bird he took it into his hands and prayed over it sobbing. Within minutes there was a fluttering and the bird regained consciousness then flew away.

John had a wonderful appreciation and love for nature and while working on his father's farm intuitively knew what was wrong with sick animals. He became known as the local veterinarian to the local farmers as he could tend to difficult calving and lambing easily with his ability to sense and see through bodies and recognised the power of silent prayer when all else failed.

His own experiences with illness have provided him with a basis for training and empathy as a healer.

He has recovered from whooping cough, measles, mumps, chicken pox, rheumatic fever, undulant fever, stomach ulcers, mild heart attack, and semi paralysis from severe back problems.

Physicians told him there was a possibility that he would never walk again unless he had a rather risky operation. This he refused, choosing instead the alternate approach of chiropractic treatment that was to him less invasive. He had seen an uncle become much worse after surgery similar to that recommended.

After two months of daily treatment there was gradual improvement and the extreme pain subsided. As the months passed he experienced gradual improvement and could get back to work.

In addition to Chiropractic he experienced acupressure, acupuncture, color therapy, vitamin and mineral therapies, hypnosis, radionics, massage, Swedish body work and manipulation, Chinese acupuncture

/acupressure and herbology, and finally Philippino Psychic surgery which alleviated the problems. His spine is now healed and strong!

Feeling there had to be more to life he studied different major church philosophies including those of the East and West, witnessed many healing sessions and developed a great interest in the esoteric fields. His special interest was in the Eastern Yogis who had developed great mind and pain control over their bodies and he read voraciously on the subject to alleviate his own pain.

Experimentation with various herbs, cell salts and large doses of vitamins and minerals was done at enormous cost with small lasting effect for him.

Next he looked into Past Life Therapy, Spiritual Releasement Therapy and remote deposessions with the Inner Peace Movement which confirmed his beliefs about what he could sense and see clairvoyantly. At this time people would say how good they felt in John's presence and what seemed like an electrical charge was often transmitted upon contact with his hands and they immediately felt better.

Another close family member became ill with no apparent medical reason so he learnt Swedish Massage and Bodywork technique to ease the situation. John studied Alpha Dynamics, a derivative of PSI, Silva Mind Control, Mind Dynamics, and other techniques and became one of the instructors, participating in their research programs and used some of their techniques for stress and pain relief.

Two renowned psychic healers from the Philippines cured his ulcers and lower back problems and a friendship developed so he was invited to show his gratitude and travel to the Philippines to work with them on a missionary basis. As at that time there were limited osteopaths and chiropractic knowledge there John's work was indispensable and he often worked from 9 a.m. to 2 a.m. the following day. He saw many miracles and his own spiritual gift and skills as a healer expanded tremendously.

After being called to India where he had three interviews, and received the blessings of SAI BABA Spiritual Leader and Avatar of India, John started the Tree of Life Healing Center in Southport, Queensland Australia, with another renowned psychic and past life therapist.

John Douglas Chamberlin is a man who walks his talk. He is a strong believer, has participated in many self-help growth seminars. He has led his own seminars in Self Healing/Past life Therapy/ Spiritual Healing/Positive Movement Bodywork Therapies/Basic Hypnosis/Leading Edge business techniques/Meditation for Stress Relief/Communication and Decision Making /Self Hypnosis for removing emotional blocks/Spiritual release Therapies/Radionics for Health and a few others.

He is also a researcher in the field of drugless medicine using natural remedies wherever possible and researching the field of radionics as a practitioner getting phenomenal results. He is grateful to universal guidance, and continues to be of service all over the world from Australia, New Zealand, United States, Mexico, Canada, British Isles, Denmark, Sweden, Germany, France, Switzerland, Philippines and many others.

He has been honoured by Prince Regent of Hutt River Province in Western Australia as Citizen of the Year 1996 and received the title of The Honourable John Douglas Chamberlin.

The power of prayer and the love of our Mother Father God/Universal energy are paramount in the expression of his healing gifts.
John feels that he is truly an instrument of God and continues to walk in the light of guidance, intuition service and love.

www.ingramcontent.com/pod-product-compliance
Lightning Source LLC
Chambersburg PA
CBHW031823170526
45157CB00001B/168